T0135640

The Cardiac Defense Response

Personality

Stress Management

Dissertation

zur Erlangung der Würde eines Doktors der Philosophie

der Universität Hamburg

vorgelegt von

Bettina Jung-Stalmann

aus Hamburg

Hamburg
2003

Bibliografische Information Der Deutschen Bibliothek

Die Deutsche Bibliothek verzeichnet diese Publikation in der Deutschen
Nationalbibliografie; detaillierte bibliografische Daten sind im Internet über
http://dnb.ddb.de abrufbar.

ISBN 3-8325-0071-5

Logos Verlag Berlin
Comeniushof, Gubener Str. 47,
10243 Berlin
Tel.: +49 030 42 85 10 90
Fax: +49 030 42 85 10 92
INTERNET: http://www.logos-verlag.de

The Cardiac Defense Response;
Personality
Stress Management

Dissertation

zur Erlangung der Würde eines Doktors der Philosophie
der Universität Hamburg
vorgelegt von
Bettina Jung-Stalmann
aus Hamburg.

Hamburg
2003

Erster Gutachter: Professor Dr. Bernhard Dahme

Zweiter Gutachter: Professor Dr. Kurt Pawlik

Abschluss der mündlichen Prüfung: 3. Februar 2001

Acknowledgements

I wish to thank Professores Kurt Pawlik and Bernhard Dahme from the University of Hamburg (Germany), Dr. Frank Eves from the University of Birmingham (UK) and the *DAAD, (Deutscher Akademischer Austauschdienst)* for being given the opportunity to do this project for a Dr. phil. in Psychology. I wish to thank Dr. Shree Balaji També, the inventor of the meditation technique used in this study for his contribution of a teaching audio-cassette specially produced for this project.

The students and staff of the School of Psychology at Middlesex University, Enfield-Site, who participated in this stressful experiment have my special thanks! The School of Psychology of the University of Birmingham is to be thanked for helping me to finish the writing up of this project by providing access to its facilities. This had been only possible because of the support of Professor David Booth and Professor Glyn Humphreys to whom I want to send special thanks for support - and teaching me some cognitive Psychology.

Dr. Derek Land, as an experienced science editor, patiently read almost all parts of my thesis, and Dr. Sandy MacRae deepened my understanding on trend analysis - very special thanks to both of them. Thanks go also to the technicians Mr. Guthry Walker from the School at Middlesex University and Mr. Manjit Singh from the School in Birmingham. Also Dr. Dietmar Heinke has to be thanked for technical advice and support. I thank him and Dr. Karina Linnell for their non-tiring encouragement and those thanks also go to Mr. David Sladen from the time in London. There are aquaintances from Birmingham University who helped me with their concern and I want to say "Dankeschön" to them too.

My godmother Dr. med. Helene Einecke and my late father Dr. phil. Reinhart Stalmann I thank for their kind generosity. Again I want to thank my spiritual guide, Dr. Shree Balaji També, for his everlasting supportive encouragement and energy that kept me going through all the difficulties.

Birmingham / Hamburg, July 2003

IV

Synopsis

The Task

This study had two orthogonal tasks based on a physiological experiment with auditory high intensity (HI) stimulation with warning and repetition. There were two experimental sessions with measurement of Heart-Rate, Skin Resistance, Electromyogram, and Respiration Rate, Subjective Measures and questionnaire data. Confirmation of the hypotheses on first session's individual heart-rate differences of the Cardiac Defense Response to the HI-stimulus and in anticipation of the impending HI-stimulus were needed as prerequisites for two orthogonal research tasks:

1. Relationship of CDR with physiologically based Eysenckian (EPI) and Pavlovian / (Strelau Temperament Inventory, STI) Personality Temperament constructs.

2. Attenuation of CDR-related reactivity in anticipation of a high intensity stimulus over 4-5 weeks of training in methods of stress management (progressive muscle relaxation (PMR) or a concentrative multimodal meditation technique, Aum Swarupa Dhyan Yoga (ASDY), and a waiting-list control group. ASDY-meditation involves chanting, visual imagery and listening to vocal / instrumental music and *Sanskrit* verses.

Dictated by circumstances allocation to the groups had to be done by self-selection. In order to take advantage of that limitation, psychophysiological differences between prospective stress management groups were investigated as well as differences between continuing and dropping–out participants.

Individual Differences of the CDR

Hypotheses on individual differences of *Secondary Acceleration* in the period of Long-Latency (15-55 sec) and a reflection of those differences in the accelerative peak of Short Latency (1-10 sec) post-first-stimulus were confirmed as well as within-session habituation post repetition of stimulus. The differences were established in response mean and response shape (operationalised by differences in linear to quartic trend- components) of *phasic* and *tonic* response to HI-stimulus replicating previous research results with similar paradigms (e.g. Eves & Gruzelier, 1984).

Individual differences of the first anticipation sequence (57.5 sec) of HI-stimulus were not confirmed. There was a tendency of individual differences in the repetition sequence of anticipation that modestly confirmed the hypothesis on sensitisation of individual differences in this sequence. The failure to confirm the hypothesis, contradicting a pilot-study, is being discussed.

Effects of Stress Management Training

Both methods contributed training effects on an adjective check-list for Mood changes. Group differences were found in the two adjectives out of 18: Meditators were more alert and less sluggish than relaxers after the introductory training session.

Synopsis

In the comparison of the two physiological experimental sessions, progressive muscle relaxation mediated response-attenuating effects on heart rate or blood pressure or on other physiological variables did not become conspicuous in comparison to the other stress management groups. It was suggested that lack of compliance was a major factor accounting for the failure to confirm the hypothesis. Nevertheless, the result seemed consistent with a previous study suggesting that success can be expected only after a training period of six months.

ASDY- Meditation seemed to have a sensitising effect on Anticipation Heart Rate of the first high intensity stimulus in the second session (but not to its repetition!) suggesting an adaptive defensive reaction to the impending physical threat in comparison to the relaxation group. The result was discussed as being consistent with research on interoception (Pennebaker, 1982) and results of an earlier study involving a different, purely cognitive meditation technique (Goleman & Schwartz, 1976).

These results have been discussed further in the light of recent research on *Pranayama* (Controlled Breathing) and its effects on the cardiovascular system.

Psychophysiological profiles of Stress Management Groups and Dropouts:

For the first time initial physiological differences between self selected groups of stress management were investigated. Prospective stress management subjects had higher sympathetic activation in anticipation of HI-stimulus repetition than controls, i.e. they were sensitised to the stimulus. There were no prospective group differences in State Anxiety and Neuroticism and this was found consistent with the dual-process theory of relaxation. Meditators using this chanting technique had more somatic anxiety than the TM-meditators of the literature who had been found to be more trait anxious than controls. Control subjects had higher resting levels of skin conductance levels and diastolic blood pressure than stress management groups and lower values in the averaged means of Anticipation Heart-Rate (of impending HI-stimulus). In addition they had reliably higher Social Desirability scores compared to both other groups. These results on lowered responsivity to physical stimuli and higher social desirability scores could be consistent with studies conducted on "impression management" given that selection of no-stress-management control group was a superb strategy to demonstrate compliance with two social demands. Participants of Stress Management Groups who dropped out of the investigation between the two experiments tended to be more neurotic than continuers. The dropouts from the meditation group were more responsive to HI-stimulation than the continuers. Hence self-selected meditators were more responsive than controls and the more responsive meditators were more likely to drop out. Hypotheses about meditation dropouts being more introvert and state anxious were not confirmed.

Relationships between Personality / Temperament and CDR

Correlations of physiologically based personality / temperament measures with cardiac defense were first tested with the criterion of presence of *secondary acceleration*. A T-test confirmed that secondary Accelerators had reliably lower scores on the scales for *Strength Of Excitation, Mobility,* And *Extraversion*, but there was no confirmation for the hypotheses on *Neuroticism, Strength Of Inhibition* at this level of analysis.

Synopsis

Direct negative correlations of test scores with the *Phasic response mean* confirmed the T-test for *Strength Of Excitation* (-0.35) and *Mobility* (-0.17) but not for *Extraversion* (-0.12). Also in line with the T-test was the negative result for social desirability. On the other hand, the response mean of short latency did confirm the predictions for *Strength of Inhibition* (-0.31) and *Neuroticism* (0.16) but was inconsistent with the T-test result.

The *Response Mean of Tonic Heart-Rate* from the sequence covering 55 seconds post stimulus was consistently negatively related to the Strelau scales, although *Mobility* was only marginal. All scales but Extraversion and mobility had reliable relationships with the resting baseline into direction of hypotheses.

Hypotheses on correlations of test-scores with the *response shape* superimposed over phasic and tonic response mean differences were also confirmed. Nevertheless, scores on *Neuroticism* were positively correlated with the quadratic component of the tonic response alone, while the response mean differences were in reverse direction. All results largely confirmed findings of a previous study by Richards & Eves (1991). Within- and between-study differences were discussed as a function of stimulus intensity and questionnaire response key.

Furthermore, significant correlations were found between the CDR and Social Desirability: resting baseline and the response shapes of phasic and tonic response mean were inversely related to Lie scores confirming an EEG-study by Kline et al (1993) about high Lie-scorers diminishing the impact of auditory High Intensity stimulation.

Table Of Content

Table Of Content

Table Of Content

1. Introduction

1.1 Introductory Comment

At the centre of this thesis are two issues in relation to individual differences of heart rate changes in response to high intensity laboratory stressors. One is covariations of those differences with physiologically based personality measures, the other is about modification of anticipatory reactivity, related to these differences by progressive muscle relaxation or an unknown complex meditation technique. A vague concept of *autonomic balance* of the two systems of nervous excitation, according to Schandry (1989) first expressed by Eppinger & Hess (1910) and Wenger (1941, 1962) was involved in the planning of this study.

Mainstream research into cardiovascular reactivity by-passed the differential aspect for pragmatic reasons by putting aside passive task paradigms as will be explained in the first section. However, the conventional differential approach, based upon a classical psychophysical interest in describing and ordering different response patterns to different stimulus strengths, carried on, and produced some results for differential psychophysiology.

1.2 In Search of the Defensive Response in Humans

Increased cardiac output is necessarily answered by a pressor-response in the vasomotor centre shunting the blood into the vessels of the skeletal musculature. This occurs in all mammals, however, the anatomical mediation is not yet clearly understood for humans (Busse, 1997). Dogs and cats for example have sympathetic cholinergic fibres leading from the cortex down to the vessels in the skeletal muscles. Perhaps beta-receptors are the responsible mechanisms as experiments with so called beta-blockers and abolishment of vasodilatation in the skeletal muscles of primates have shown (Schramm, Honig & Bignall, 1971). The cardiovascular regulation system in the medulla together with the vasomotor responses in the peripheral system (skeletal muscles, inner organs, and skin), mediated by the catecholamines from the adrenal medulla is regarded as the main physiological expression of the defensive response in mammals. The function of the response is to put the organism into a state that facilitates intensive action: an emergency reaction as the pioneer in this research area wrote (Cannon, 1915). Metabolic changes in liver and spleen add to this preparatory function.

The response can be elicited by stimulation of some points in the limbic system and those studies are amply described in the literature and were reviewed by Shapiro (1982). One can find there e.g. that Hess (1949) used the term defensive reaction (*Verteidigungsreaktion*) for the first time for the behavioural pattern of a conscious cat in response to electric stimulation of the posterior thalamus. The pattern was described by initial alerting followed by flight or attack. Abrahams (1960) then stimulated identical points in the posterior hypothalamus of an unconscious and a conscious cat and thereby produced evidence for the direct relationship between these particular points, increased

CO, the reciprocal vascular changes in skin, viscera and skeletal muscles, and co-ordinated defensive behaviour in the conscious cat.

While the behavioural pattern can be described quite clearly for dogs and cats each with species-specific features, this issue is not clear at all for the human behaviour. This is because our social environment does not allow us to exert the behaviour for which the physiological response pattern has just prepared us via the hypothalamic-sympathico-adreno-medulla mechanism in response to aversive stimuli in the environment (Schandry, 1989). The physiological reaction without its behavioural counterpart has long been regarded as a potential cause for disease (ibidem). Particularly, increased cardiac output (CO), a function of heart rate and myocardial contractility, that is not used for exercise has been regarded as the main initiating cause of hypertension in genetically predisposed individuals (Folkow, 1982, Obrist, 1982).

Folkow was inspired by the first study describing the physiological defensive response by Brod, Fencl et al (1959) with ten normotensive and eight hypertensive human subjects. They measured cardiovascular responses to *mental arithmetic* with harassment. Most subjects showed increased CO and forearm bloodflow during stressor-impact and decreases in the *splanchnic* area. Four subjects across both groups had decreased CO and instead increased peripheral resistance that led to increased heart rate (that was not documented). This difference between "cardiac" and "vascular reactors" to stresses is an example of individual-specific-reaction (individualspezifische Reaktion, ISR, Schandry, 1989) and that will be discussed in the next paragraph. Until today cardiac output is not easily accessed and the merit of this study is that this important variable was measured by invasive methods [1] and that thereby the hemodynamic pattern which the human and animal organism produces during exercise occurred in context with stressful mental arithmetic. Moreover, that pattern measured in humans under stress was reminiscent of the fight or flight response in animals.

This result was several times confirmed by studies with inventively varying forms of harassment. However, later studies skipped the variable harassment and the reactions became smaller in magnitude but not different in quality. Mental work like word-association testing and mental arithmetic *per se* seemed to be linked to the cardiovascular pattern of the defensive response with pressor-response to cardiac output and vasodilation in the skeletal muscles. No psychological threat that could have affected the *posterior* hypothalamic area was needed to put the subjects into an exercising like state.

Obrist (1976) then drew attention to the behavioural component of the defensive response by manipulating the subject's activity in the experimental design, calling it *active* and *passive coping*. He had proposed that both heart rate and somato-motor activity were integrated by the central nervous system (CNS) explaining acceleration and deceleration of the heart rate as a consequence of somato-motor behaviour. This theory of cardio-somatic coupling integrated a number of studies on directional fractionation of the heart rate. The approach implied that no particularly stressful stimuli were needed to elicit metabolically unnecessary, exaggerated cardiac output in certain individuals. Obrist produced convincing evidence for his hypothesis, by presenting differential cardiovascular response patterns for the active/passive-coping variable. His main tool of evidence was pulse wave velocity in

---

[1] CO and blood pressure were taken from arterial and venous points in the arm and injected dye was traced in bloodsamples

Introduction – In Search of the Defensive Response in Humans

the carotid artery (carotid dp/t), an indirect measure for cardiac output, as well as heart rate and systolic and diastolic blood pressure (SBP, DBP). When activity was required during experimentation such as shock avoidance tasks, playing video games or mental work, blood-pressure control was more dominated by cardiac influence. In contrast, when passive endurance of events without any possibility of avoiding the impact of the stressor by increased motor activity was required, as with cold-pressor test or a pornographic film, blood pressure control was dominated by vascular influence. The hedonic/aversive aspect was added in order to have more control over the activity-variable. Obrist's evidence was impressive because the pattern of changes from baseline in all three vascular variables were reversed in active and passive coping tasks. Carotid dp/t, systolic blood pressure (SBP) and HR were reliably more elevated from baseline values while diastolic blood pressure (DBP) hardly changed in the active reaction time tasks. Conversely, DBP indicating vasodilatation and therefore no constriction in the peripheral resistance vessels (going along with increased cardiac output) showed greater changes in the passive tasks. Carotid pulse wave was the best discriminatory variable although the validity of this variable is not given at between-subject level because calibration is not possible (Schandry, 1989). However, the interaction with the other variables was impressively consistent with Obrist's hypothesis. The active-coping paradigm also allowed identification of the more reactive subjects, i.e., the potential hypertensives, and so research on cardiovascular reactivity was now carried out almost exclusively with active-coping tasks, unless vascular reactivity was meant to be the variable under investigation. The only passive coping stressor was the cold-pressor test, but high intensity stresses were not investigated in this context – most probably because these paradigms are ethically not easy to defend and lack therefore user-friendliness for both investigator and potential subjects.

The dichotomy of active versus passive coping also integrated other results from animal as well as from human-research. Two cats were studied in confrontation, preparation for and during a fight with each other. During the fight, both cats developed the physiological fight/ flight response pattern as expected. However, the preparation period while flinching, retracting ears, dilating pupils and watching the adversary, was marked by vasoconstriction in the hind limb muscle, and by decrease of cardiac output and deceleration of the heart rate (Adams, Bacelli, Mancia & Zanchetti, 1971). Subsequently this pattern was labelled as "immobile confrontation" by the last author. Also the directional fractionation of the heart rate as a function of sensory intake and sensory rejection (Libby, Lacey & Lacey, 1973) then suggested muscle vasoconstriction for the former and dilatation for the latter.

In the same paper that introduced Obrist's new paradigm of active coping - it was a presidential address to psychophysiological colleagues in 1975 - he dismissed purely stimulus-response oriented research into cardiovascular reactivity without involvement of the behavioural component. He proposed that any *phasic* (within 15 s) changes in HR would occur due to somatic activity, e.g. postural changes, because the myocardium was predominantly under vagal (parasympathetic) control, namely inhibited as soon as the organism started becoming physically active, which was known as the *exercise effect*. Only tonic (>15s) accelerative changes from baseline in response to a stressor could be appreciated as sympathetically driven. These would occur in an experimental context with specific coping-demands such as a task with a handicap wherein 25% subjects showed exaggerated HR-accelerations of 40 beats per minute (bpm) in comparison to the average who showed only 24 bpm. Therefore these active coping paradigms offered more opportunity to understand how the "stresses of life contribute to cardiovascular disease" (p.104). He also admitted that individuals would respond tonically to "more passive stresses" (ibidem) and that will be taken up later in the chapter.

The active / passive coping paradigm is not quite without flaws. Mental work does not fit into the category of active coping because there is a mediating link between cognitive activity and somato-motor behaviour. Besides, does not, for example, a passive coping situation with a highly aversive stressor come closer to real life stress situations than an active coping paradigm because there is no option of attack or escape for most events in professional or private life? This is at least what life event research suggests. Obrist (1982) argued that tonic sympathetic influences on the myocard were observable only in active-coping paradigms where "some control over the stressor" was given as well as novelty; this contrasts with paradigms of classical conditioning (passively waiting for an unavoidable stressor). He found that intensity of the stressor was difficult to operationalize and his own studies on intensity were inconclusive.

The classic methods originating from psychophysics and analysing psychophysiological stimulus-response relationships, continued to be in use by investigating which physiological and stimulus parameters actually discriminated the defensive response from the other major response pattern crucial for survival of the species, the *orienting response*. Finally, a third pattern, the *startle reflex*, had to be considered. The first step of all scientific research is the need for exact description and classification of the phenomena under investigation. The classic approach proved firstly the *dominance of heart rate* for discrimination for the time being and secondly discovered *tonic sympathetic effects*. Thirdly *individual differences* were found since not everybody in the population responded with these tonic sympathetically induced accelerations of the heart rate to stimuli of high auditory intensity.

1.3 The Acceleration of the Heart Rate as a Marker ...

The Cognitive Origin of Orienting and Defensive response

It was in the late twenties when studying the conditioned response that Pavlov (1947) discovered a response pattern fundamental to the survival of the mammal, the *orienting response* (OR). Sokolov (1963, p.545) quoted his teacher's classical definition from his work on the orienting response, understood as a reflex at the time.

> "It is this reflex that brings about the immediate response in man and animal to the slightest changes in the world about them, so that they immediately orientate their appropriate receptor organ in accordance with the perceptible quality in the agent bringing about the change, making full investigation of it. The biological significance of this reflex is obvious. If the animal were not provided with such a reflex its life would hang at every moment by a thread. In man this reflex has been greatly developed in its highest form by inquisitiveness – the parent of that scientific method through which we hope one day to come to a true orientation in knowledge of the world around us." (1, p.27)

Sokolov had continued Pavlov's work with physiological experiments on low, or moderate stimulus intensities thereby focussing on the movements of the bloodvessels. In his article on "The Orienting Reflex" (1963) he described *cephalic vasodilatation* together with a generalised activation pattern in responses to low and moderate stimuli and in contrast, *cephalic vasoconstriction*, in responses to higher stimulus intensities. Sokolov believed that vasodilation facilitated *neural sensitisation* and thereby integration of the new stimulus environment, namely via correction of a mismatch between a neuronal model of known stimuli and the novel stimulus. Vasoconstriction of the brain vessels, in contrast, desensitised the system thereby limiting the impact of the stimulus. While the former response pattern was Pavlov's Orienting Response (OR), the latter was now given the name *Defensive Response* (DR). Turpin (1983) explained that Sokolov's interest was actually psychophysical, (i.e. quantification of how physical stimuli are psychologically experienced) and not psychophysiological, (i.e. how physiological changes are psychologically experienced), which might have narrowed his perspective. His concept of the OR was actually entirely based on an approach of cognitive neuroscience and applied exclusively to novel stimuli. The EEG was the method most referred to in the paper and heart rate was dismissed as a component of the orienting reflex by referring to animal literature of the time on responses to acoustic background stimuli (p.546/47)

"… thus such changes of heart rate cannot be regarded as components of the orienting reflex".

Graham & Clifton (1966) inferred from this passage and an earlier article that for Sokolov "heart rate accompanies orienting" (p. 306) and referring to his article on "Perception and the conditioned reflex" of the same year they concluded that for Sokolov in general, increased sympathetic activity seemed to have an excitatory and facilitating effect on cortical activation.

The Lacey's however demonstrated at the time with experiments with complex stimuli that this was not true for increased heart rate and blood pressure and came up with their concept of *environmental intake* expressed and facilitated by heart rate deceleration and *environmental rejection* by heart rate acceleration (1964, cit. Graham & Clifton). The Lacey's suggested that vagal activity indicated by the deceleration of the heart rate enhanced cognitive processing and that this function occurred *intentionally* and not as a reflex. In spite of this "ideological" difference (raising a debate between Elliott (1972) the Laceys (1974) and Obrist, Webb *et al.*, 1970) the Lacey's environmental intake-rejection concept functionally meant the same thing as Sokolov's *neural sensitisation*. But while their crucial variable, the *fractionation of the heart rate* determined intake and rejection, Sokolov's were constriction and dilation of the bloodvessels in the brain.

Graham & Clifton (1966) in their review settled the matter by stressing that studies reporting heart rate acceleration as part of OR had in fact elicited a DR or a startle, and thereby suggested a third generalised pattern elicited by *fast stimulus rise-times* (see below). They concluded that only paradigms with *non-signal stimuli* (e.g. series of tones of low intensity without information content) had elicited deceleration and hence the environmental intake enhancing OR. The third criterion to discriminate between the two was habituation: OR habituated quickly with repetition and DR did not.

Acceleration of Heart Rate in Short Latency and Startle

Graham & Clifton (1966), Graham and Slaby (1973) and particularly Graham (1979) reporting her work on the effects of stimulus intensity and acoustic stimulus rise-time to its full strength, indexed the response patterns by direction of the heart rate changes.

Deceleration characterised OR and acceleration during the period of short latency (1s-10s) post-stimulus became "the heart" of the DR. Also, Raskin, Kotses & Bever (1969) confirmed with a study of differences between the two patterns. Stimulus intensity, heart rate and skin potential response discriminated between the patterns but vasomotor changes did not. Turpin & Siddle (1978) suggested that Sokolov presumably had worked with the long latency response (see below) and therefore had found cerebral vasoconstriction. Graham & Clifton had already stressed that cephalic vasodilatation had not been found consistently with OR but sometimes with DR. Besides: the cephalic bloodvessels were as difficult to assess as heart rate was an easy option. All those facts together led to heart rate becoming the main dependent variable to discriminate between the OR and DR.

However, a new problem had to be dealt with from now on: Startle (SR) manifested with "a unique skeletal muscle pattern of widespread flexor contraction" also occurred in those ten seconds post-stimulus onset and acceleration of the heart rate might have been part of this system (Graham, p.149). Graham and Slaby (1973) tried to avoid the dilemma of two confounding systems by separating cardiac startle from cardiac defense at the second post-stimulus second. The argument was that startle was only elicited with fast rise-times and habituated with stimulus repetition whereas defense could be elicited with both slow and fast stimulus rise-times and did not habituate. Sokolov also had assumed the DR to be resistant to habituation.

However, Turpin & Siddle (1978) used slow rise-times with high intensities and found the elicited response habituating with repetition. They suggested therefore the response of the short latency period and its habituation as a function of behavioural startle (widespread muscle flexion) which was a function of the energy properties of the stimulus, being determined by such factors as bandwidth, intensity and rise-time. By further questioning Graham's evidence for startle, occurring within the first post-stimulus second, they suggested that differentiating between the two components should cease.[2] Because of these problems of differentiation between cardiac startle and cardiac defense, the heart rate acceleration of the short latency period cannot be considered a suitable marker of the DR.

Secondary Acceleration in Long Latency Period, Fight or Flight Response

Turpin & Siddle (1978) experimented with several presentations of a 110dB white noise stimulus and found a secondary acceleration of the heart rate in the period 10s to 70s post-stimulus with a peak at 30s. The only problem was that the pattern disappeared with stimulus repetition. The authors suggested that this secondary acceleration of the heart rate was the true cardiac part of the defensive response by presenting three pieces of physiological evidence for a link with the fight or flight response in animals.

They found an increase of forearm girth, measuring bloodflow and indicating distribution of blood away from the inner organs to the skeletal muscles. Secondly, negative changes of ECG T-wave amplitude had suggested sympathetic activity caused the acceleration of the long latency period but not for the short latency period (however, the validity of this measure is not undisputed). Thirdly: a study on the fight or flight response

---

2 In a more recent study Turpin (1992) presented evidence for risetime and intensity as effecting physiological and behavioural startle with the notion that also slow risetime together with low intensities could do.

in dogs and cats (Bond, 1943, cited in Turpin & Siddle 1978 and in Eves & Gruzelier, 1984) reported accelerations of the heart rate in both latency periods with the same temporal characteristics. Ablation studies by the same author had shown evidence that the secondary acceleration resulted from sympathetically mediated release of adrenaline, while the first short latency acceleration may have been caused by both vagal inhibition and increase in sympathetic tone. Graham & Clifton (1966) by referring to Obrist, suggested that the acceleration linked to *vagal inhibition* occurred due to the "respiratory gasp" or larger inspiration with stimulus on-set (p.313). They referred to the same mechanism known from respiratory sinus arrhythmia (RSA), the complex influence of the respiratory cycle on variations of the heart rate, which in some cases can be clearly observable in a parallelism of respiratory and heart rate "curve" recorded by the polygraph (the latter as displayed by the cardiotachometre). The inhalatory phase promotes acceleration while the exhalatory phase slows the heart rate down. This phenomenon has been partially ascribed to *inhibiting* impulses fired by the stretch receptors in the lung to the afferences of the *vagus* reaching the inhibitory heart centre in the medulla (e.g. Schandry, 1989). The vagus is a major player in the parasympathetic system e.g. by slowing down heart-rate via acetylcholine application on the sinus node.

More recently, i.e. after the experimental works for this thesis had been already completed, Reyes & Vila (1993) investigated experimentally that larger "respiratory gap": In fact the inspiratory cycle increased with stimulus onset regardless of the phase (inspiratory or expiratory) in which the stimulus was presented. That was because expiration turned into inspiration when the stimulus was presented then and therefore the authors termed that process "inversion of the expiratory phase" (p.23). They concluded that the first acceleration could have been a result of respiratory sinus arrhythmia, the inhibition of vagal activity caused by firing of the inspiratory neurones, stimulation of lung inflation receptors and stimulation of the lung inflation reflex by changes in blood pressure linked to respiration (see Reyes & Vila for references). However other findings about decrease of RSA mean amplitude in the same study presented elsewhere (Reyes, Godoy & Vila 1993) suggested rather a centrally mediated parasympathetic withdrawal instead. Regarding the secondary acceleration these authors found increase in breathing amplitude linked to its elicitation and suggested the secondary acceleration being for a part a consequence of hyperventilation with CO_2 level reduction, potentiation of sympathetic responsivity and inhibition of vagal cardiac activity. A more recent study on physiological variables associated with the response pattern to high intensity stimulation in collaboration with G. Turpin (Perez & Fernandez et al., 1999) also suggested lesser vagal mediation during second acceleration in long latency than in short and more sympathetic participation instead promoted by vagal cardiac inhibition. The authors suggested the existence of complex sympathetic-parasympathetic interaction for the whole response pattern termed the Cardiac Defence Response, (CDR) which in this thesis will be spelt in the American manner as it is always found in the databases: Cardiac Defense Response.

The study mentioned last continued the research on individual differences of the CDR which was started by Eves (1984, 1985) following Turpin & Siddle's earlier findings that eventually had linked Sokolov's defensive response to another mammal survival mechanism, the fight or flight response.

1.4 The Cardiac Defense Response and Individual Differences

Confirmation of CDR and Discovery of Individual Differences

In a series of three experiments with intensities from 112-127 dB tone Frank F. Eves (1985) found two types of heart rate accelerations in his studies for a Ph.D. The first occurred in the short latency period (1-10s) the second in the long latency period 15-50s post stimulus onset (Eves & Gruzelier, 1984). All subjects showed increases in forearm girth and digital pulse amplitudes in both periods of latency, indicating enhanced skeletal muscle bloodflow and vasoconstriction in the skin. This was some evidence for blood redistribution from the inner organs and the skin to the skeletal musculature (Eves & Gruzelier, 1987). However, there were individual differences across all intensities and the proportions varied. Firstly: More than half of the subjects showed no heart rate acceleration in the long latency period and, in contrast, a considerable number of them showed heart rate deceleration. Secondly: The number of subjects showing secondary acceleration increased with intensity from 112dB but then remained constant from 122 to 128dB.

In order to quantify the between-subject differences a non-parametric procedure was applied. The criterion for secondary acceleration was that during the long latency period significantly more heart-beats fell into the bandwidth of > 4 bpm above baseline than < 4 bpm above baseline (*Accelerators*). Conversely, deceleration in the crucial period was defined by having a significant majority of heartbeats falling into the category < 4 bpm below baseline (*Decelerators*). There was a third category of subjects not falling into either category; they were named *Equivocals* suggesting the main character of their HR-changes. By application of this procedure, the author found in the second experiment with 127dB tone in a sample of 25 medical students on average 43% secondary Accelerators, 29% Decelerators and 28% Equivocals. In two other experiments with four different samples the proportions varied between 40 and 45 for Accelerators, 28 and 36% for Decelerators and 14 and 30% for Equivocals. There were no baseline differences between the three subgroups and there were no differences in the subjects' ratings of aversiveness and loudness of the high intensity tone. The heart rate sequences of the two latency periods related to the baseline and the polynomial contrasts were then analysed with multivariate analysis of variance, which confirmed significant differences between secondary Accelerators and Decelerators in both latencies. The individual differences of the long latency period were not linked to any differences in Startle as shown by analysis of cardiac acceleration of the first two seconds post-stimulus to baseline and movement artefacts in the ECG. Accelerators and Decelerators were different in magnitude of the accelerative peak (2-4s) in the period of short latency, and in the quadratic trend component of this period.

The differences of the long latency period, however, habituated with stimulus repetition as Turpin & Siddle already had established. Therefore, the author concluded, in contrast to Turpin, that the long latency response could not have been the basis of Sokolov's observation. Dishabituation of the DR had been Sokolov's second differential criterion for OR and DR. However, there was a third sequence differentiating between subgroups additional to the two in long and short latency post-stimulus: In the period of warning of the impending high intensity stimulus 55s before onset, the subgroups were different in the quadratic trend component. However, there had been decreases in T-wave amplitude at linear and quadratic trend level for both subgroups indicating that both groups were activated via the sympathetic system.

The differences between the two subgroups were interpreted as resulting from different evaluations of the acceleration of the short latency period. The author suggested that secondary Accelerators were perhaps similar to "less behaviourally restrained subjects" from an early study on startle from the thirties, who simply ran away in response to the stimulus (see Eves & Gruzelier for reference).

Physiological Mechanisms - the CDR as a Homologue of the Fight or Flight Response

Animal studies with ablations of the adrenal medulla had produced evidence that the secondary acceleration was a result of the catecholamines elicited through the hypothalamic-sympathico-adrenal-medulla system, circulating in the bloodstream and speeding the heart rate through its various electro-chemical effects on the heart-muscle (Schandry, 1989, Jaenig, 1997). The question was, which mechanism did account for the deceleration in the long latency period. Again ablation studies on animals, namely on baroreceptor inhibition after hypothalamic stimulation (e.g. Lisander, 1970), suggested an explanation. The baroreceptors are stretch receptors most frequently distributed in the carotid sinus artery in the neck and in the aortic arch next to the heart-muscle reaching with their fibres directly to the cardio-inhibitory centre, or to a nucleus in the medulla. The receptors "fire" in response to increase of pressure in the aorta and thereby inhibit tonic discharge of the vasoconstrictor nerves and excite the cardio-inhibitory centre. This mechanism lowers systolic blood pressure and makes heart rate decelerate. The defensive response depends on baroreceptor inhibition and the authors suggested that the Decelerators had no baroreceptor inhibition after the short latency response.

> "In short, while high intensity stimulation may reflexly produce sympathetic-adrenal activity in both groups, for Decelerators the blood pressure control systems operate unhindered. In contrast, Accelerators, inhibiting baroreceptor modulation of cardiac rate, exhibit the true defensive response." (Eves & Gruzelier, 1984, p. 350-51).

The authors also suggested that the secondary acceleration indicated the readiness to limit the stimulus behaviourally by escape or fight and the Accelerators thus would exhibit the "true defensive response" (p. 351). Further evidence for this assumption was taken from minor cardiac subgroup differences in forearm girth (Eves & Gruzelier, 1987). As mentioned above, in both latency periods all subjects had increased bloodflow in the skeletal musculature. However, the cardiac subgroups differed reliably in the quadratic and cubic trends of the long latency period. The changes in secondary Accelerators' were indeed closer to a quadratic trend, whereas the Decelerators' changes showed a significant cubic trend and thus were decelerative. Turpin & Siddle (1978) and Turpin (1983) had presented these concomitant events of heart rate and bloodvessel changes earlier. However, these trend differences were not to be underestimated because the forearm girth signal indicates not only blood flow in the skeletal muscles but also in the cutaneous vascular beds and therefore the signal underrated the muscle bloodflow (Heistad & Abboud, 1974). Hence there was enough evidence to link defensive response and fight or flight response closely together and for the claim that only less than half of the population show the defensive response in laboratory experiments with high intensity stimulation.

1.5 Individual Differences of the CDR and Personality

1.5.1 Extraversion and Neuroticism - The Eysenck Personality Inventory

Overview

The bipolar dimensions of Extraversion (E) and neuroticism (N) are trait theoretical constructs, orthogonal to each other and based on some physiological assumptions on differential processes of reception and processing of sensory and emotional information in the central nervous system. The Maudsley Personality Inventory (Eysenck, 1959) was the first standardised questionnaire to assess psychometrically these dimensions. The Eysenck Personality Inventory (EPI, 1963) represents an improved version of the MPI containing a control instrument for answering biased by social desirability, the so-called Lie-scale. It measures the tendency to respond to self-evaluative questions in a socially approved manner in order to appear more attractive to others or to him/herself. The Eysenck Personality Questionnaire (EPQ, 1973) was expression of a further development in the authors personality theory by supplementing a third dimension named psychoticism. The following section will provide the theoretical and empirical background to the scales of the EPI and the presentation is mainly based on Eysenck & Eysenck (1985) and Eysenck (1967).

Trait - Theoretical Background

Traits are dispositions or tendencies of an individual to behave consistently across time and situations in a particular variety of ways to a definable range of stimuli. Thus an extravert person would tend to respond with a "typical" outgoing behaviour in social gatherings while an introvert person would most likely respond with equally typical shyness. In fact, those traits interrelating with each other constitute the personality types as primary factors load on secondary factors. The primary factors of Extraversion are described by the (bipolar) adjectives sociable, lively, active, assertive, sensation-seeking, carefree, dominant, surging and venturesome. The primary factors of Neuroticism are anxious, depressed, guilt-feelings, low self-esteem, tense, irrational, shy, moody, and emotional. Therefore these types should not be misunderstood as fixed categorical concepts like the four temperaments (sanguine, choleric, melancholic and phlegmatic) by the antique physician Galen. Every person can be described by a position in the four quadrants described by the two orthogonal dimensions Extraversion and Neuroticism.

Some Science Historical Roots

It was Wilhelm Wundt who inspired Eysenck's concept of Extraversion rather than Carl G. Jung who seems to have the copyright to the term. That is because Jung's concept was based rather on assumptions of individual differences in processes of drive (libido) and subconsciousness than of differences in the central nervous system. Wundt, in contrast, had explained Galen's four temperaments as a function of *strength and speed* of change in a person's feelings. Hence both sanguines and melancholics were seen as "weak" in affect, cholerics, and phlegmatics as "strong." While sanguines and cholerics had a fast rate of emotional changes, melancholics and phlegmatics took a rather slow pace of emotional change. One can see that Wundt had transformed Galens four categorical types into an infinite number of individualities localised in a plane described by *emotional strength and changeability.*

The noun emotionality deriving from the Latin word for feeling is today often preferred to the term neuroticism (e.g. Fahrenberg, 1991) and it seems indeed a more behaviourally correct descriptor for Eysenck's concept as his physiological assumptions will show.

A Neural Network as the Agent of Personality Differences

A system of neurones in the medulla because of its network-like structure named *formatio reticularis* is responsible for wakefulness of the organism. Earlier it was believed that the somato-sensory afferences in the medulla would stimulate the cortex but unequivocal evidence showed that stimulation of the ascending reticular activating system (ARAS) evoked desynchronisation of the EEG (Moruzzi & Magoun, 1949). Further evidence from lesion studies showed that the somato-sensory afferences running parallel to the reticular formation in the brain stem functioned as its collaterals when cut off above the medulla oblongata. There are circuits of excitation, or loops, from the ARAS to all subcortical locations and to the thalamus from where excitation is directed to the cortex. Whether there are direct pathways from the reticular formation to the cortex is not unequivocally reported by different physiological presentations. While Carlson (1991) was in favour of such direct connections Birbaumer & Schmidt (1997) were not. However, there was no dissent on Eysenck's hypothesis that individual differences in the cortico-reticular loop itself accounted for differences in Extraversion. More extravert individuals has less tonic activation in the reticular system while the introvert is chronically more activated. Therefore both seek a different stimulus environment: The extravert goes predominantly for environments high on stimulation, the introvert looks predominantly for the opposite.

There is a second loop with collaterals from the limbic system, Eysenck named it the "visceral brain," to the reticular formation which "fires" then up to the cortex (that would then be the "limbic-reticular-cortical loop"). While the cortico-reticular loop is empirically established and can be found in the textbooks under physiology of wakefulness, a connection between visceral brain and reticular formation is only implicit. Such a loop exists but Eysenck (1967) noted that the significance of the reticular system could be over estimated in this context because the hypothalamus has its own activating functions by direct cortical connection and by its autonomic activities which in turn activate the reticular formation (footnote 2, p.232). Either way, differences of activity in the limbic system (hypothalamus, amygdala, hippocampus, cingulum and septum) predominantly linked to emotions in the literature, accounts for differences on the N-dimension. Individuals high in Neuroticism (or emotionality) would produce more activity in the limbic system than less neurotic (emotional) individuals.

Evidence for Eysenck's Hypotheses

The cortico-reticular hypothesis found a considerable body of confirmatory evidence. Introverts showed slower habituation times to the orienting response and the majority of studies with depressant and stimulating substances, e.g. alcohol and caffeine, showed reliable differences confirming the hypothesis. Depressants reduce activation of the reticular system, which is why introverts become "extraverts" under alcohol influence. Stimulants increase cortical activation, which is why extraverts reverse their normal inferiority in vigilance performance tasks after caffeine while introverts remain unchanged. Also white noise has improved extraverts' abilities on this task. Also Pavlov's law of *transmarginal inhibition* could be demonstrated as being consistent with the construct of Extraversion. The law says that a nerve cell's excitability increases with stimulus intensity but goes into transmarginal inhibition when the threshold for sustenance is reached. Introverts are naturally expected to have lower thresholds than extraverts. Several studies were conducted the most simple of which worked with auditory stimulation of 80 dB and 100dB. The results showed introverts having higher SCL than extraverts at 80 dB but the differences reversed at the higher intensity. The introverts had reached their inhibitory threshold before or at 100dB.

There was only contradictory evidence concerning the "visceral brain-reticular-cortical-loop" hypothesis. Fahrenberg (1991) argued for retention of the null-hypothesis on the basis of multivariate and multi-situational studies of his own (1987), and others and particularly of Myrtek (1984). That was consistent with Eysenck (1967) explaining that the stress levels of "our type of society" would rarely be strong enough to make people reach "a state of fight or flight in the meaning of that phrase given to it by Cannon" (p. 233). The distinction between activation caused by sensory input (he called it arousal) and emotional stimulation would only break down "in a very small proportion of the population and under unusual circumstances, e.g. in war" (ibidem).

Eysenck & Eysenck (1985) defended the hypothesis against the contradictory evidence in habituation studies of OR (N slows habituation speed) by making methodological flaws responsible for some of the negative results. According to their review, skin conductance does not indicate differences of habituation rate but finger volume responses do. Inconsistencies of results from stress research were put down to stressor inadequacy. "The problem may Lie in the persistent use of insufficiently stressful conditions" (p. 234). Fahrenberg (19912) reserved the possibility of predictable physiological differences between high and low emotional or neurotic subjects for "highly stressful conditions" but considered it as unethical to investigate those in the laboratory.

However, Richards & Eves (1991) had been interested whether biologically personality measures could predict presence or absence of HR-acceleration in long latency, i.e. measures independent from the stimuli used to elicit the response. Among others, they put Eysenck's hypothesis to the test. They found evidence by T-test for Accelerators scoring reliably higher on N than non-Accelerators (Decelerators and equivocals collapsed). Further, by application of analysis of covariance they found the test scores covarying positively with heart rate at several levels of measurement: Resting baseline heart rate and mean heart rate suggested high scorers having higher tonic levels. Relationships with response-shapes were also found: High N-scorers showed a more pronounced quadratic trend, superimposed over the response mean, in the period of long latency. The response mean of the short latency period covaried with N too in the same direction but there were no reliable trend-differences between high and low scorers. Fahrenberg's null hypothesis was challenged.

Similar results were achieved with the scores on Extraversion. This time the relationship was inverse: Accelerators were more introvert than non-Accelerators at T-test level and introverts (low scorers) had higher baselines, a higher response mean in both latency periods and a more pronounced quadratic trend in the period of long latency, superimposed over the response mean.

Social Desirability and Cardiac Responsivity

The problem of questionnaire data is whether people respond in honesty to the questions. The problem with honesty is that individual truthfulness collides with social pressure, which in behaviourist terms is called *social desirability*. In order to control that bias in his questionnaire, the Lie-scale was added to the EPI. According to Eysenck & Eysenck (1975) it does not only reflect simple "dissimulation" but also a stable personality factor linked to "social naivety." However, recent research suggested differences in physiological responsivity between low and high Lie-scorers.

Social desirability is a moderator variable in all the research fields relevant to health: stress, personality, psychopathology and to critical epidemiological investigations. That is because denial of undesirable behaviours can lead researchers to attribute a disease to other factors (see Brody, Veit & Rau, 1997 for reference).

Some investigations found cardiac reactivity positively related to Lie scores on Eysenck scales. College students with high Lie scores showed greater HR responses to a live assertive response situation than low scorers did (Kiecolt-Glaser & Greenberg, 1983). In addition, experimenter-advised mental arithmetic (MA) tasks showed high HR-reponsivity related to Lie scores. Brody, Veit *et al* (1997) had no such differences in a computer-advised MA task suggesting that for participants high on social desirability the results be moderated by the interaction with the experimenter.

Social desirability scores have often been interpreted as *defensiveness*: Jamner & Schwartz (1986) found that high defensive subjects (EPI, Lie) had higher pain thresholds and were more pain tolerant than medium and low defensive subjects, measured by self reports, but had no higher sensory thresholds. It was well possible that these results were moderated by "high impression management" though, i.e. conscious denial of weakness. However, the same first author (Jamner, Schwartz & Leigh, 1988) later found immunological evidence for high Lie-scorers being repressors at the physiological level. They had immunological profiles typical of a high degree of central opioid tonus and both studies were consistent with the hypothesis that repressive coping is related with diminution of the impact of intense or painful stimuli.

Kline, Schwartz *et al.* (1993) used parameters of the EEG to test the hypothesis whether high defensive subjects (EPQ, Lie) repressed incoming moderate and high intensity tones at cortical level. They found smaller auditory evoked potentials (lower amplitude intensity slopes) at intense stimulus levels (94db, 104dB) but not at moderate level (74dB, 84dB). This may suggest the hypothesis that Lie scores covary negatively with cardiac responsivity to high intensity auditory stimulation and perhaps reversely that non-Accelerators score higher on Lie than Accelerators.

1.5.2 Pavlov's Strength of the Nervous System - The Strelau Temperament Inventory

Strelau's Temperament Inventory (STI) originates from his collaboration with the *Moscow School* led by the Pavlov student Teplov and his own student Nebylitsin. It was the most influential of the Russian, or say Pavlovian schools, because of a systematic psychophysiological methodology for experimental assessments of individual differences of temperament in the laboratory. The term Temperament generally implies *innatedness* of the concept quite in contrast to the term personality that does not make implications of that kind. Two significant Pavlov students have questioned the temperamental status of the concept but their arguments were "convincingly" refuted by Teplov, as Strelau remarked (1983, p. 24).

A Sanguine Dog as a Nervous System Type

The STI is developed on the basis of observed behaviour but its theoretical basis stems from Pavlov's "nervism" which postulates that any behaviour is governed and regulated by the central nervous system. It was conceptualised on the basis of his conditioning research with dogs and was continued and developed further by his pupils' work with human subjects. The section is almost exclusively based on Strelau's book on "Temperament, Personality, Activity" (1983) starting with the beginnings of Pavlov's theory:

> "Systematic observations of the behaviour of dogs, during experiments on classical conditioning, led Pavlov and his students to the conclusion that there exist strongly expressed individual differences in the speed and accuracy with which both positive and negative (inhibitory) conditioned reflexes are elaborated in their efficiency, strength and durability, in the ease with which they may be changed and, finally, in the manner in which animals behave in the experimental chamber." (Strelau, p. 1)

Pavlov postulated the existence of *two* antagonistic mediating *brain processes*: one to *excite* and one to *inhibit* responses[3] and ascribed further the basic properties of *strength and equilibrium (balance)* to these two processes. Later he added a third property, *mobility*, which related to the speed of change between the two processes. Variation in these properties "moderating" the brain processes of excitation and inhibition accounted for individual differences and particular configurations of these variables constituted certain types that were identical with the ancient characters by Galen. In fact, Pavlov often referred to two descriptions of his laboratory dogs as representatives of Galen's types. His student

---

[3] Eysenck (1987) called Pavlovs theory a proponent of arousal theory. As a matter of fact the very first draft of his personality theory (Eysenck 1985) was even based on the assumption of differential excitatory and inhibitory processes in the reticular formation. Extraverts e.g. had more inhibitory processes inbuilt and introverts less and the latter were therefore chronically more aroused and so on. This concept did however not work experimentally and so he "reversed" the concept to the described activation theory, called arousal theory in those days before directional fractionation of arousal had been implemented in psychophysiological theory.

Nikiforowsky (1910, cited in Strelau, 1983) had made them celebrities of scientific history in his Ph.D. thesis and they should be honoured here as they were by Strelau (1983).

" (1) ...The type with predominance of excitation over inhibition. These dogs are sensitive and mobile, they do not behave quietly during the experiment, and the smallest changes in the experimental situation evoke strong expressed reactions;

(2) ...The type with predominance of inhibition over excitation. Dogs belonging to this type do not usually change their posture during the experimental procedure and their reaction to unexpected or unusual stimuli is slight. Evoked conditioned reflexes become very quickly inhibited;..." (ibidem p.2)

The first dog reminded Pavlov of the *sanguine* and the second one of the *melancholic* type. The former was regarded as *strong, balanced* and *mobile*, the latter as *weak*. He drafted his own typology along the three properties but worked out only the strong side: The phlegmatic was seen as strong and balanced like the sanguine but with slow speed of change and the choleric was regarded as strong but imbalanced. Hence, Pavlov had chosen a deliberate combination of the constituents that would have produced logically at least 24 types as he admitted (ibidem p. 6). Pavlov's little obsession with Galen's types (he insisted that all his dogs could be put into these categories as Strelau wrote) must be forgiven with regard to his lucid conceptual neurophysiology and its experimental operationalisations in the laboratory. That classification system was published in 1925 (General Types of Higher Nervous Activity in Animals and Man) and became the basis for the work of his students.

i.   Strength of Excitation: That is the "working capacity of the nerve cells."It materialises in the "withstanding of either prolonged or short-lived, but exceedingly strong, excitation without slipping into protective transmarginal inhibition (see previous section). The strength of excitation can be estimated by recording the organism's responses to strong, prolonged, or recurrent stimulation" (ibid. p. 3). Strength of excitation is described in this operational context as a state. The term has indeed both meanings of state or trait and depends on the context. State means the level of the excitatory process at a particular moment and that depends at least on three variables: *intensity* of the stimulus; *tonus* of the cortex or level of *activation* dependent on fatigue, hunger or other variables, and the *property* underlying individual differences in the strength of excitatory process evoked under constant maintenance of intensity and activation. Consequently, the strength of excitation was investigated by manipulating the first two variables. The stimulus intensity limit was found at which adaptive responses could be evoked or the activation level was increased pharmacologically or by food deprivation. Additionally the speed of CR-acquisition and durability was measured by determining the number of UCS presentations and of CS presentations without reinforcement for extinction. A dog with a strong excitatory process needed only few UCS presentations for acquisition of the CR and kept them stable. "Dogs with weak processes would need longer to develop a CR and that would lack stability over multiple CS-presentations.

ii.   *Strength of inhibition*: There is no clear definition in Pavlov's work. Nevertheless, he was "referring to conditioned acquired inhibition" (Strelau, p.6) when he spoke about this property of the nervous system. Hence, it is the capacity to build up and to maintain an inhibitory conditioned response. There was a further complication in the development of this operationalisation: In Pavlov's first concept the weak type had well developed inhibitory conditioned responses and low strength of excitation and was therefore named the inhibitory type. Later he changed his view. The weak type was considered low on both dimensions. The weak type shows low conditioned internal inhibition but is characterised by strong unconditioned external inhibition (Strelau, 1983, p 6).

iii. *Balance or equilibrium* relates to balanced occurrence of both processes.

iv. *Mobility* as the third property is "the ability to give way - according to external conditions - to give priority to one impulse before the other, excitation before inhibition and conversely" (Pavlov, 1952, cited by Strelau, p. 9). "...Mobility manifests itself by the speed with which a reaction to a given stimulus, when required, is inhibited in order to yield to another reaction evoked by other stimuli, etc.; the environment is continuously changing, therefore the individual, in order to adapt to these conditions, must modify his nervous processes in line with these changes" (ibidem).

Research on Humans: Strength and Sensitivity

It is clear that the *strong type* understood as trait shows weaker excitatory responses under stimulating conditions while the excitatory states are enhanced in the weak system. It is therefore not difficult to conceive that the strong type can be identified as the extravert in Eysenck's system and the weak type as the introvert. Gray (1972) modified Eysenck's theory by "relocating" the degree of Extraversion from activity in the ARAS to a particular area in the limbic system involved in responses to reward and punishment (frontal orbital cortex, medial septal area and hippocampus). Therefore, he used Introversion as reference term rather than Extraversion. There is evidence from animal studies that stimulation of the hippocampus inhibits the ascending pathways of the ARAS to the thalamus and Gray assumed therefore a negative feedback loop formed by the septal hippocampal ARAS system which accounts for differences in Introversion. From here, he inferred the possibility that the dimensions of Introversion and strength of the nervous system are in fact identical. Particularly the mechanism of protective transmarginal inhibition, central to the Russian concept, "is due precisely to the operation of the kind of feed back loop discussed here as the physiological basis of Introversion" (ibidem p. 192, see also Gray, 1964).

Teplov and Nebylitsyn concluded that strength of excitation could be regarded as a bipolar dimension with *endurance* at the one end, where from strength of excitation had been assessed following Pavlov's methodology, and *sensitivity* on the other (Strelau, p. 29). Hence strength of excitation could be assessed from the sensitivity pole and that seemed to have solved the ethical problem of having to use high stimulus intensities. They were needed to determine the threshold to transmarginal inhibition that marked the limit of strength. Pharmacological stimulants enhance excitation capacities of the cells, therefore application of a caffeine dose lowers the sensitivity-threshold, and normally supra-threshold stimulus intensities will become detectable. The dosage needed for such changes provides then the measure for sensitivity.

The Partiality Phenomenon

However, having solved the ethical problem the next "troublemaker" walked in through the backdoor: the *partiality phenomenon*. Ivanov-Smolensky, another student of Pavlov had discovered through his work on conditioning motor reactions with hundreds of kindergarten and school aged children that the measures of nervous system properties were highly dependent on the modality the unconditioned stimulus belonged to. In addition, the type of reinforcement influenced the categorisation of the properties. Nebylitsyn elaborated the partiality phenomenon systematically and tried to get control of it by assuming independent functional circuits serving different purposes, perceptual and regulatory. However, the works of other Russian researchers stated that there were far more sources for partiality causing discrepancies in the investigation of nervous system types (Strelau, p 50). Strelau himself worked on the problem and found that the partiality problem was even "much broader than has been stated by Nebylitsyn and can definitely not be limited to the inter-modality differences stressed by that author" (ibidem p. 115). "Discouraged" he turned to methods "which are not concerned with psychophysiological reactions or laboratory conditions but which are aimed at diagnosing Nervous System Properties on the basis of more molar behaviour" (ibidem).

Human Behaviour and the Properties of the Nervous System

Strelau translated the physiological construct of the nervous system properties into terms of human behaviour as follows:

> ➢ Strength of excitation (StE) into: "ability to do long lasting and intensive work, speed of recovery after fatigue and intensive activity, persistence and ease in coping with obstacles";

> ➢ Strength of inhibition (StI) into: "ability to regain control, ability to refrain from given activity, restrained speech";

> ➢ Mobility (M) into: "ease of passing from one activity to another, ability to organise behaviour in situations requiring different kinds of activity, uninhibited social contacts"(ibidem, p 116).

Relationships with other Physiologically based Constructs

StE is as a psychometric construct related to Extraversion (e.g. Richards, 1986; Daum & Schugens, 1986). A minor number of papers reported no correlations between the two scales (e.g. Stelmack, Kruidenier & Anthony, 1985). While Richards & Stelmack et al. used a forced choice answer scheme - yes / no - Daum & Schugens used the three-response format with a "don't know" option as in Strelau's original questionnaire.

Relationship with the Cardiac Defense Response

The same study that was introduced in context with the EPQ (Richards & Eves, 1991) could show that inverse relationships exist between the CDR and test scores on Strelau's StE and StI scales. Accelerators achieved reliably lower scores for both scales than non-Accelerators and low StE and StI-scorers had reliably higher heart rate response means in both post stimulus periods of latency. The pre-stimulus baselines were also affected by the covariance factor and that suggested tonic differences between low and high scorers. There were phasic differences reflected in covariations with the quadratic trend component of long latency: Low StE and M scorers had a more pronounced quadratic trend superimposed over the response mean differences.

Based on the reactivity hypothesis the authors regarded their results as being relevant to the prevention of primary or essential hypertension because of the link of excessive cardiac output to the defensive response. Their results also contributed to evidence for the hypothesis on the physiological basis of Personality. They referred to a similar link between electrodermal responsivity and the STI reported by Strelau (1986).

1.6 Clinical Relevance of the CDR: Phobia and Hypertension

Physiological changes accompanying phobic reactions with the defensive response pattern had already been established and the secondary heart rate acceleration with phobics in response to confrontation with phobic materials was added by Sartory, Eves & Foa (1987). Eves, Blizard *et al* (1990) provided some evidence that a hereditary factor is involved with long latency acceleration of the heart rate by hierarchically modelling the between-subject and within-subject variance of dicygotic and monocygotic twin pairs with regard to genetic and environmental factors.

The acceleration of the heart rate in the period of long latency has been explained as a consequence of differences in baroreceptor control of bloodpressure that facilitated the preparation of the organism for fight or flight. This suggested higher levels of state anxiety, but evidence for that hypothesis has not yet been found in the previous studies about the cardiac subgroups (Eves, 1985).

Some publications have brought the defensive response into context with development of essential or primary hypertension. That is because it is known from the beginning of research of the matter by more than a hundred years ago that hypertensives have a hypertrophy of the left cardiac ventricle and thickened aortic and arteriolar walls (Folkow, 1990). It was as early as 1877 that these hypertrophies were suggested to be a consequence of "raised pressure (tension) in the vascular system 'uebermaessige Spannung im Gefaess-System'" and the author even hinted at "hemodynamic consequences" (Ewald, 1877, cit. Folkow, 1990, p. 90). For reasons of methodological research limits and of "fads and fashions" of research task selection (ibidem), the idea of structural adaptation of the vascular system to raised peripheral resistance was followed not before the second half of our century. Folkow (1982) developed a theory based on his own experimental evidence and application of hemodynamic laws. He suggested that heightened systemic resistance in the arteriole vessels stem from structural alterations in the vascular walls and consequently "upward structural resetting" of human hypertensive resistance vessels. There are two environmental factors in Folkow's model influencing these changes: heightened bloodflow results from salt intake habits and/or "certain excitatory psycho-emotional influences." A necessary condition for these factors coming into effect is the hereditary predisposition of the individual. Folkow (1982), inspired by a study on the defensive response to a forced mental arithmetic task (Brod, 1959) particularly considered the defensive response habit in mild and strong variations as such psycho-emotional influence.

Obrist (1982) linked increased cardiac output (a function of heart rate and contractility, both effected by sympathetic activation) to development of elevated peripheral resistance.

Forsyth (1971) had observed bloodpressure four times in monkeys during a 72-hour shock avoidance task. In the first measurement, cardiac output was elevated and in all three subsequent measurements, peripheral resistance had increased. This is one of several experiments, which indirectly supported the *reactivity hypothesis* on development of hypertension.

The linking of hypertension and phobias to the defensive response led to the assumption that reactivity associated with this reaction should be sensitive to treatment with methods of Stress Management.

Clinical Relevance of Attenuation of CDR related Reactivity

There is another line for cardiovascular disease prevention linked to modification of CDR-related reactivity: Fifty percent of sudden cardiac deaths occur in persons with no previous diagnosis of ischemic heart disease (Fraser, 1986). The hearts of many sudden death victims show scars of old infarcts and it has been questioned that always myocardial infarction precedes sudden death (ibidem). Then ECG abnormalities such as premature ventricular contractions and particularly "a pattern of fine, focal *myocardial fibrosis*"[4] (ibidem p. 200) play a dominant role in the pathogenesis of sudden cardiac death. One variety of focal myocardial lesions was linked to catecholamine-excess. Also the "disturbances of the sympathetic nervous system arising from acute stress can apparently alter the *ventricular fibrillation* [5]threshold". Since therapy *post-lethal* infarct is not possible, prevention is particularly important. If this thesis could confirm Eves & Steptoe's results on direct attenuating effects of progressive muscle relaxation on cardiac reactivity in a longer term then the method could be recommended for those risk patient with myocardial fibrosis in their ECG.

---

4 thickening of muscle with connective tissue
5 uncoordinated writhing of the ventricular heart-muscle fibres

1.7 The CDR and Methods of Stress Management

1.7.1 Progressive Muscle Relaxation

Progressive muscle relaxation (PMR) as a self-regulation method has been shown effective in reducing autonomic activity as documented in reviews (e.g. Borkovec & Sides, 1979), although the pathways of those processes are not yet well understood. The rationale is that by relaxing singular muscle groups in several training sessions "generalisation takes place to other muscle groups, and to situations outside the laboratory" (Steptoe, 1989, p.223f). However, "though a number of studies have shown EMG reductions at specifically trained sites during relaxation training, the literature suggests that generalisation to the skeletal musculature in its entirety is hard to achieve" (ibidem).

According to Lehrer (1982) and Lehrer, Batey *et al.* (1988) the inventor of this procedure, Jacobson, asked his patients to perceive the tensions and to relax one muscle area after the other progressively in long lasting sessions up to 2-3 hours. Today an abbreviated method has been introduced by Bernstein & Borkovec (1973) and is widely used in clinic and laboratory. The client is asked first to tense deliberately particular muscle groups and then to release the tension. This is progressively done with gross muscle groups throughout the body. The rationale is that firstly the client learns to attend to the feelings of tension and of relaxation that occur as a consequence of those procedures. Secondly it is assumed that after high tension the muscle relaxes deeper which is understood as a *pendulum effect* (Bernstein & Borkovec, 1973) "The clinical goal is to increase the clients ability to identify even mild tensions and to efficiently eliminate that tension. This newly acquired skill can then be applied to maintain low levels of physiological activity during the day in general and in response to environmental stresses in particular" (Borkovec & Sides, 1979, p.119).

However, general muscle tonus is very difficult to measure because none of the particular muscle sites is an indicator for general tonus and the correlations between the different muscle groups are poor (Steptoe, 1989).

Reduction of Tonic Activity

Borkovec and Sides (1979) reviewed 25 studies on physiological effects of progressive muscle relaxation training. The studies were classified according to whether progressive relaxation was found superior to appropriate control conditions in reducing physiological arousal, or equivalent, or inferior to those conditions. Fifteen studies showed superiority of PMR over control conditions. The two groups of studies differed significantly in number of sessions and live vs. taped instructions. More training sessions (4.57) was superior over fewer (2.3), and therapist administration was superior over taped instruction. The groups tended to differ on the employment of patient vs. normal samples. In those studies which showed superiority of PMR over control conditions the proportion of clinical against normal samples was 7: 8 (47%) whereas in the group "PMR equivalent or inferior" only two (20%) out of ten studies employed clinical samples. Thus statistically, relaxation applied in multi-session by a therapist to populations concerned with physiological hyper-activation will have the best prognosis for success in physiological activation reduction. The overlaps of both groups do not exclude non-clinical samples (seven among the 15 successful studies had normal subjects, but among the 10 unsuccessful studies, only two had clinical samples), using taped instruction.

Looking at the different physiological variables measuring activation, three studies using normal populations reported cardiac reductions (Beiman, Israel et al., 1978; Brandt, 1973; Paul, 1969) during or after relaxation. The same studies reported reductions in the EMG, as did Reinking & Kohl (1975) and Schandler & Grings (1976). Changes in galvanic skin resistance (GSR) frequency were reported by the authors first mentioned and by Green, Beiman et al. (1977). Delman & Johnson (1976) and Paul (1969) reported changes in respiration.

Reduction of Stress-Induced Responsivity

There are a few studies investigating the effects of relaxation on responsivity to threatening situations. Some studies were successful, others not. Kirsch & Henry (1979) reported reductions of cardiac activity in speech anxious subjects following desensitisation with PMR. Heart rate was assessed before giving a speech, once before training and once after three weeks training. The subjects treated with PMR showed reliable reductions of response heart rate, whereas the competing methods, meditation and no training, showed no effect. However, in another experiment with a stressful situation (Boswell & Murray, 1979) subjects were told they had performed poorly on an IQ test and a digits backwards test. Two-week relaxation training had no effects. Puente & Beiman (1980) reported reductions of heart rate elicited by aversive slides after cognitive restructuring combined with PMR. One of the competing methods, behaviour therapy combined with self-relaxation, was successful in reducing heart rate.

A more recent study (Blanchard, McCoy et al, 1988) on 73 hypertensive subjects compared PMR thermal biofeedback and drug withdrawal as potential substitutes for sympatholytic antihypertensive medication. They measured blood pressure and heart rate in response to three stressors (mental arithmetic task, cold pressor, negative mental imagery) before and after training. Reductions were found more for PMR than for biofeedback and more for mental arithmetic and systolic blood pressure. Craske & Rachman (1987) could show direct effects of PMR on cardiac responsivity in a mixed-age group of anxious musical performers after four weeks of training in PMR and attention focussing. All subjects had reductions of fear (subjective report) and a high heart rate group (by median split) had reduced their anticipatory heart rate. At a three-months-follow-up measurement, those who had return of fear had also increased heart rate thus suggesting that PMR can reduce arousal in certain kinds of threatening situations if therapeutic interventions are combined with PMR.

There were four experiments using threatening stimulation with loud acoustic stimuli but none of them reported cardiac reduction effects: After four weeks of training Lehrer et al. (1980) found no differences between PMR and a waiting list control group in heart rate accelerations to five loud tones (100 dB). The experimental subjects were anticipating the tones while practising the method they had been trained in. Cardiac accelerations as measured by the difference between pre- and post-tone-maximum heart rate did not give rise to any group differences. There were no differences in either EMG or skin conductance. The same author reported similar results three years later: no differences in cardiac accelerations but the PM group produced bigger decreases in the forearm EMG.

The third study using aversive acoustic stimulation (Brandt, 1973) reported attenuation of baseline for EMG and heart rate but no effects of PMR on reactions to aversive tones.

Modification of CDR-related Reactivity by PMR

Eves & Steptoe (1987/89) investigated the effects of brief training (48 hours) in progressive muscle relaxation (PMR) and heart rate biofeedback (HBF) on the dis-habituating subgroup differences in the warning periods of an impending high intensity auditory stimulus. For response elicitation and dis-habituation, they worked with a stimulus combination of high intensity white noise and preceding moderate intensity warning with two presentations. The exposures to the stimuli were interspersed by a 90s interval for recovery. Heart rate (HR), skin conductance (SC), and electromyographic activity (EMG) of the neck musculature (measuring startle) were recorded as physiological (dependent) variables. On the basis of the first session's heart rate recordings the subjects were post-hoc categorised into two subgroups, according to their cardiac responsivity in long latency and by means of the procedure laid down earlier by Eves & Gruzelier (1984) explained in the previous section. Secondary Accelerators formed the high reactive subgroup, secondary Decelerators and Equivocals formed under the name non-Accelerators the low reactive subgroup.

After the first laboratory session, subjects were assigned to one of three conditions: Jacobsonian progressive muscle relaxation (PMR), heart rate biofeedback (HBF), and control. The subjects of the former conditions received either one live training session of 30-49 minutes PMR or instructions in the use of a prototype ambulatory biofeedback instrument plus ten minutes training. The subjects of the control group remained without training of any kind. PMR was then practised twice daily for thirty minutes along with an instruction tape. The biofeedback instrument could be used in two modes: one working with a continuously present tone in the earphone another with a tone in 'threshold-mode'. The frequency of the tone in the former was related to their heart rate, in the latter the tone was audible only when heart rate was 15 bpm above baseline assessed in the laboratory. The subjects were suggested to use the threshold mode during their daily activities and additionally they had to engage in a 30-minutes period of practice with the continuous tone during each day in order to enable themselves to control their heart rate.

The laboratory experiment with the paradigm of repeated presentation of the stimulus combination and recording of physiological responses was repeated 48 hours after the first experiment and training session. The departmental paper of the Eves & Steptoe study did not make clear whether there was a relaxation sequence before the resting period. Only "two periods of voluntary HR control" after the resting period were mentioned (p. 11). Otherwise, there is no mention of any practice during the experiment.

As expected from the previous studies, the individual differences of the long latency period habituated with repetition within the first session. As also had been predicted, the subgroup differences were reflected in the warning period: the Accelerators showed higher responsivity than the non-Accelerators during both warning periods. Therefore, treatment effects would be particularly sought in the warning periods of the second session.

Univariate analysis of the heart rate baselines revealed that the Accelerators had elevated baselines in the post treatment session. Skin conductance levels were unchanged across sessions but the Accelerators had reliably higher resting levels overall. There were no differences at any level in the baseline data of the EMG indicating that cardio-somatic coupling did not account for the session differences in heart rate.

Analysis of responsivity post-stimulation showed Accelerators in the control- and HBF-group exhibiting higher levels of HR than the subjects from the low reactive subgroup during all 4 periods of the second session at overall mean level. In contrast, in the relaxation condition, the mean subgroup differences after relaxation training occurred only following the first warning stimulus of the second session. The Accelerators' first anticipatory augmentation of heart rate had not been abolished but the differences overall and the second anticipatory augmentation had. The anticipatory sensitisation effect in the first session was easy to accommodate within the classical conditioning theory but the anticipatory effects of the second session in HBF and control group were regarded as unusual and needed explanation.

The authors regarded the methodological features of the paradigm as crucial for the effects, i.e. brief exposure to the unconditioned stimulus (UCS) and a "protracted intercession interval." They had found similar features in paradigms used in studies on aquisition of behavioural avoidance and cardiovascular anticipatory changes in primates. The authors explained further the underlying processes for the anticipatory sensitisation effect as a particular form of classical conditioning – context dependent learning between conditioning sessions - and alternatively as paradoxical enhancement. The treatment effect of PMR training was accommodated within the two alternative explanations:

Firstly: Learning needs peripheral sympathetic activity for memory modulation. Thus, the relaxation training may have interfered with the process of memory consolidation between sessions. Secondly: The relaxation training developed a competing response in the experimental context. However, that does not explain why the PMR-Accelerators augmented their heart rate in response to the first warning.

There were effects of training on Accelerators for both treatment groups in the EMG-data of the neck muscles in response to high intensity, reflecting startle. For Accelerators in both the relaxation and HR-feedback conditions, reactions were clearly attenuated in the second session, whilst in the control group the elicited EMG changes were similar to those in the first session, particularly the response to the first stimulus. For the relaxation-group, the absence of individual differences and attenuation of response were neatly consistent with the HR data because the rationale for PMR emphasises treatment effects on the skeletal musculature. However, the effect in the biofeedback group questioned the whole issue, for the rationale of HBF does not involve such direct effects at all. The authors therefore offered two alternative explanations for the HBF-effects on startle: Either the practising of reducing heart rate had a generalised effect of "somatic quietening" or rapid habituation had taken place in this group within the 48 hours of inter-session interval. This was possible because the gross motor components and the associated muscle potentials habituate rapidly in contrast to peripheral contractions like eye-blink (Landis & Hunt, 1939; Davis, 1948, cit. Eves & Steptoe). The question following the latter explanation was why the control group had clearly dis-habituated to the first stimulus but not to the repetition stimulus. Because of the controls' habituation to the repetition stimulus, the authors considered habituation could have happened in all groups. Nevertheless, the startle reflex to the first stimulus of the second session was as well developed as in the first in the control group, even the repetition response was a rather clear-cut peak in contrast to the startle profiles in the treatment groups. The authors eventually discussed the result in the relaxation group in context with a cross-sectional study that had produced a similar effect of PMR on startle (Lehrer, 1980) free from confounding habituation effects. From this result and from the fact that tonic reduction effects had not occurred they inferred reduction of activity in the neurological pathway for startle. They described this effect as similar to that of anxiolytic medication. They also regarded the startle reflex as a potentially "useful addition to the more commonly monitored physiological variables in treatment of anxiety states" (Eves & Steptoe, 1987, p. 21). The effects of relaxation were also accommodated within both alternatives by the authors: "...relaxation training following the experimental session could be expected to interfere with the process of memory consolidation, for it should preclude the elevated peripheral sympathetic activity which has been associated with memory modulation. Alternatively, training in relaxation would involve the learning of a competing response within the experimental context"(ibidem).

The skin conductance data showed no evidence of training effects. Instead, similar levels of activity in Accelerators occurred throughout both sessions, also with a reduction in levels across session for the less reactive subjects. The lack of differential effects was put in context with the weakness of subgroup differences in the first session. Furthermore, a dissociation of SCL and HR seemed to be more common for the CDR than an association: Out of four studies, only one had shown SCL as a concomitant variable. In studies with hypertensives and phobics, such dissociation had also been demonstrated.

On the one hand the results of Eves & Steptoe had replicated individual differences in the long latency response (to high intensity auditory stimulation in humans) and rapid habituation of these differences. On the other hand, they had added evidence in support of two other hypotheses:

Firstly: dis-habituating responsivity and that is understood as reactivity, related to the differences of long latency, namely in the preceding anticipatory periods of warning. That is, paradigms with high intensity auditory stimulation and preceding warning in a passive-coping paradigm would discriminate high cardiac reactors from low reactors.

Secondly: brief training in muscle relaxation could abolish these differences in cardiac reactivity. The former had been brought forward by Eves (1985); the latter was the most direct evidence for attenuation of cardiac reactivity that had been presented before.

1.7.2 Meditation

The Roots of Meditation Research: A Central Response

Therese Brosse (1940) who was interested in the ability of a highly experienced practitioner of meditation to bring his heart rate down to zero undertook the first study into effects of meditation. Such abilities of Indian ascetes have been reported and have to be seen in a specific context of their training to become independent from physical environment in order to achieve spiritual freedom. Wenger & Bagchi (1961) found one yogi who could perspire by raising his body temperature within 1 ½ to 10 minutes. He had aquired this skill with hard practice over a long period of time by visualizing himself sitting in a hot environment in order to be not disturbed in his meditation. He had lived for some time in a cave in the Himalayas where temperatures could sink down to 0^0 Celsius. In a normal environment his efforts had the result of getting into a state of perspiration. These abilities were easily explained as a result of conditioning. They could also explain Brosse's findings of zero heart rate as a measurement artefact, however, bloodflow back to the heart had been markedly reduced in Wenger & Bagchi's study too due to physical impact from a particular exercise combination involving abdomen, breath and glottis typical of *hatha* yoga practice (p 315). This manipulation also displaced the heart and caused an effect of zero heart rate in lead I, which was Brosse's only lead in her study.

Although effects of meditation on heart rate are central to this study such efforts to achieve a certain control over the autonomic nervous system have little to do with what western meditators would want to accomplish *(see criticism of Holmes review)*. What is central are the possible psychophysiological changes enabling abilities to cope with stress, for example *Accelerators* among meditators to respond rather more decelerative when anticipating a threatening stimulus than Accelerators among control subjects without such training. Reductions in heart rate changes and other autonomous parameters as effects of meditation practice have been investigated along with concomitant changes in brain rhythms. The first studies on meditation of this kind were undertaken between 1955 and 1961 and are interesting because they were not all consistent in their results. This has been "glossed over" in the past by declaring the inconsistent results as artefactual as will be shown.

The electroencephalogram (EEG) was for a long time the only method to reveal anything about central responses to the centrally active stimulus meditation. The EEG-research is being reported and the Ganzfeld theory of meditation effects introduced before the results on peripheral autonomous activity are reviewed. In that context also a critical review of research on meditation by David Holmes (1984, 87) will be discussed.

There is the expression "someone is in meditation". It could mean that someone is in a particular mental state that he or she has achieved to get into by using a meditation technique, which he or she has been trained to use. There is a great number of different meditation techniques from different cultures and a short overview and categorisation are subject of the next section.

Techniques and Definitions of Meditation

Naranjo & Ornstein (1972) have ordered meditation techniques by two categories: *concentrative* and *mindful*. Concentrative is a meditation technique that uses an object to concentrate or to dwell upon. The object can be external like a lotus, a cross, or a presentation of a geometric shape, or internal like the visualisation of objects, reciting or chanting of a litany, a short prayer, a word, or a syllable. A speciality of yoga meditation, various internally generated sounds, *nadam*, is use of e.g. humming or high frequency sounds. It can also be the sound of a bell ringing or a sound of a flute - like imitations of other instruments (Ornstein, 1972, p. 133). In fact, one of the different yoga-systems uses sound as meditation object. Sound in Sanskrit is a synonym for the supreme level of consciousness - *nadabrahma* - because of its potentially powerful effects on the nervous system facilitated through specific sound qualities and compositional structures (També, 1981).

The term *mindful* usually applies to Zen techniques which intend to open up and expand the mind instead of focussing by allowing all contents without evaluation to enter the mind and to pass by *like clouds* as a common metaphor would describe it. Zen philosophy stresses the expansion of the mind. Zen techniques usually consist of sitting with open eyes and counting breaths or gazing at a white wall (*see EEG- section*). Another common Zen technique is listening to sounds of a waterfall; even thinking of a *koan*, a paradox phrase like the famous *sound of one hand clapping*. The mindful techniques are seen as "non-directive, in which the person lets himself be guided by the prompting of his own deeper nature" (Ornstein, p.133). The concentrative meditation techniques are seen as a "directive approach to meditation in which the individual places himself under the influence of a symbol" or holds on "to a rigid form handed down by tradition" (Naranjo, p.15). He stressed that the symbols develop their own specific dynamism by being themselves representatives of a "higher consciousness" "… evoke their source and lead the meditator … to his deepest self" (ibidem).

Naranjo (1972) made a superficial differentiation that has become a basis for categorisation in research. He attributed freedom of the mind wrongly to *zen* techniques alone. To allow anything that comes to mind "letting pass like a cloud" and then return to the mantra without being rigid, is just the other side of the coin of mantra meditation. He seemed having misunderstood *yogic* "technology" as restrictive when he quoted Patanjali, the Vedic author on Yoga, who described the function of *yoga* as *the inhibition of the modifications of the mind*. The Hindu tradition simply has a greater wealth of techniques, among them also counting own respiration rate or heart rate. The aim of meditation techniques and yoga- exercises is to expand awareness by transcending the culturally and socially mediated restrictions of sensory perception common to all societies.

Ornstein (1972) referred among others to a classic of western philosophy, Aldous Huxley, to describe the "reducing valve" function of the brain (p.171). In order to transcend these culturally induced limitations of perception, a discipline is needed for the body by exercising it in specific ways. That is because, according to Patanjali (Krishnamacharya, 1974), the central nervous system can be used to control those modifications, (or distractions or agitations) that prevent most people from living a creative life. That would be a life that would be conceptualized rather by their own design than external stimulation (see next section).

It is anyway difficult to see the difference between concentrating on a syllable or concentrating on respiration-rate or on a certain patterns of movements. Another branch of meditation techniques are movement-meditations such as *whirling* practiced by Islamic mystics, or *Tai Chi*, a Chinese form coming from the martial art tradition. The martial arts themselves, like kung-fu, can be also regarded as meditation techniques because the movement patterns of the exercises are strictly prescribed and designed by monks not only for self-defensive purposes but probably also to achieve changes in mental states.

Jevning, Wallace & Beidebach (1992, p.415) defined meditation for the "purpose of their review" quite narrowly by making the often achieved subjective result the purpose of a meditation technique. According to that very limited definition meditation is a

"stylized mental technique from the Vedic or Buddhist traditions repetitively practiced for the purpose of attaining a subjective experience that is frequently described as very restful, silent, and of heigthened alertness, often characterized as blissful."

Goleman & Schwartz' (1976, p. 457) presented a definition of meditation that may include all active forms of meditation but excludes popular beliefs of meditation as "ruminating on a conceptual theme". It is

"... the systematic and continued focusing of the attention on a single target percept ... or persistently holding a specific attentional set toward all percepts or mental contents as they spontaneously arise in the field of awareness." It is "per se ... the self-regulation of *attention*, not of belief or other cognitive processes"...

or as Austin (1998, p.92) put it more recently:

"Meditation training ... is teaching a person how to reach – and hold on to – one or several abilities to *attend*." (Emphasis not included).

A well-known story from the Zen tradition may confirm the latter authors from the side of the masters of meditation.

"One day a man of the people said to the master: 'Master, will you please write for me some maxims of the highest wisdom?'

Ikkyu immediately took his brush and wrote the word

'Attention.'

'Is that all'? Asked the man. 'Will you not add something more?'

Ikkyu then wrote twice running:

'Attention. Attention.'

'Well,' remarked the man rather irritably, 'I really don't see much depth or subtlety in what you have just written.'

Then Ikkyu wrote the same word three times running:

Attention. Attention. Attention.'

Half angered, the man demanded: 'What does that word 'Attention' mean anyway?' And Ikkyu answered, gently: 'Attention means attention.' " (Quoted from Ornstein, 1971, p.142).

Giving importance to attention as one of the major cognitive abilities, interestingly, is not unique to the teachings of meditation. Attention has been taken as identical to consciousness throughout the cognitive science debates of the nineties. But that has been unique to the teachings of cognitive science.

Problems of the EEG Method

Fenwick (1987) at the beginning of his review pointed out the limitation EEG measurements have and he regarded it as a blunt instrument for detection of brain activity in relation to behavioural variables. The EEG signal is generated by synchronous thalamic activity (modulated by the activating reticular system) to the cortex and picked up by scalp electrodes at commonly specified sites. The EEG rhythms derive from synchronisation of large pools of cells ($6cm^2$ of coherent activity are estimated to be necessary to be seen in the recordings) and thus their appearance reflects only diffuse regulatory processes, in other words local resolution is pretty bad in contrast to temporal resolution. Artefacts coming from eye movements are difficult to control since the frequency range of the EMG is very broad covering most of the EEG bands (Hugdahl, 1995). The EEG rhythms are not specific to behaviour according to Fenwick, Schandry (1989) takes a more lenient position.

Austin (1998) a neurologist and experienced practitioner of *Zazen* in one gave a detailed critical and balanced account of the research body. Meditative states are complex, there is no such thing as one meditative state but a series of dynamic changes within a subject, and there are individual differences between subjects as well. He summarized the research results in terms of EEG-rhythms within three stages, which meditators of different techniques have been found with during meditation. The first stage is an increased amount and amplitude of *alpha*. At the second stage *theta* was found being predominant some of which was consistent with drowsiness but also of short bursts and some over longer periods with increased amplitudes. Bhuddist chants – a very active form of meditation technique, interestingly, was also found associated with enhanced rhythmic synchronous *theta* activity. The third stage that some experienced meditators may show are low voltage fast beta-ripples superimposed upon still slower waves.

Fenwick (1987) with his more sceptical perspective, earlier on, had denied the EEG rythms *any* specificity. He mentioned that alpha activity would not only appear in a relaxed state but also in coma just before death and faster frequencies of (>20Hz) may be indicative for an analysing mind as well as for *coma vigile*, a condition when there is no response to any sensory stimulus. He also mentioned that "numerous examples" of the biofeedback literature would demonstrate the same changes of cerebral rhythms as long-term meditation practice (p. 116). Austin (1998) confirmed, however, quoted a study that denies biofeedback methods the subjective experience of *kensho,* the zen equivalent of enlightenment in its different varieties (Kiefer, 1985, cited as in Austin).

The early interest in meditation or: the ARAS and the teachings of Patanjali

Psychologists took their first interest in the psychology of meditation from a neurophysiological perspective. Moruzzi & Magoun's (1949) discovery of the activating reticular formation and its responsibility for wakefulness had been challenged by reports from India that highly proficient practitioners of *yoga* could reach a mental state of heightened consciousness called *samadhi*, in which they were oblivious to external and internal environmental stimuli, although their higher nervous system remained conscious. The first three studies on effects of meditation (Das & Gastaut, 1957, Bhagchi & Wenger, 1957 and Wenger & Bhagchi 1961; Anand, Chhina & Singh, 1961) consequently were studies on such highly experienced meditators following the path laid down by the Vedic author Patanjali (about 500 B.C.). The claimed insensitivity of the yogis was in a wider sense consistent with Patanjali's model of the relationship between mind, body and consciousness, a practical application of *sankya* philosophy (e.g. Honderich, 1995, entry: Indian Philosophy). In all three studies *samadhi* is treated as a central variable, but the term has more than one meaning for Patanjali and therefore in the Indian tradition. In two of the studies the stage of *samadhi* had been subjectively achieved but in which sense the term was used remained in the dark. Therefore a short excursion to the classic source of yoga teachings is being made here. Furthermore: except for the authors of the first two studies not much has been written about these basics of yoga philosophy in the papers that dealt with the investigations of its practice. However, it is appealing from a cognitive science point of view since it contains a comprehensive theory of perception and consciousness.

The following paragraph relies entirely on an introductory textbook on yoga philosophy by Malhotra (2001) who presented Patanjali's 196 sutras for the first time in plain English.

Yoga comes from the *sanskrit* syllable *yuj* implying "a union or an assimilation of two seemingly different entities". Yoga in this context means "the union of the essential self of a human being with the essence of the universe" (p.4) and this is the popular interpretation of the etymology of yoga. Malhotra has provided another interpretation deriving from the opposite content of *yuj* and gave an elucidating explanation of the Vedic model of the mind/body-consciousness relationship: *Yuj*, namely, also implies "disunion of seemingly similar entities" and

> "...according to this interpretation a human being is a combination of a material organism and pure consciousness. The everyday, 'average' existence, where each human being is trained and conditioned to accept and conform to arbitrary linguistic distinctions, social, cultural and scientific values as well as personal likes and dislikes, leads one to accept one's bodily and mental existence as the only reality. One thinks of consciousness as a by-product of biophysical processes. The aim of yoga is to help each human being to break these barriers of language, society and personal idiosyncrasy. Yoga provides a step-by step procedure to dismantle the fetters of these conditioning elements so that the individual may realise the separate existence of one's reality, which is pure consciousness. Once the individual grasps that he is essentially pure consciousness, different and separate from psychophysical processes, he is disunited from his false notions. At the same time the individual is also united in his thoughts, feelings, emotions and actions to his real self "(Malhotra, p4).

Yoga, according to the second sutra of the first chapter (*samadhipada*), "is stilling of all mental fluctuations" (1.2) and Patanjali goes on to explain "When the fluctuations are completely silenced the seer experiences one's true self as a witness to the world" (1.3). However, so the third sutra tells "When they are not stilled, an individual identifies one's true self with these mental fluctuations" (1.4). The fluctuations are categorised and explained in the next six sutras and they are five and "both painful and not painful": "correct knowledge, error, fantasy, sleep and memory" (1.5 - 6). He suggested the yogi should after a phase of physical and mental purification from disturbances (illness and fluctuations of the mind) and meditation practices, start the ultimate task of yoga, which is total withdrawal of consciousness from the senses by transcending the attraction of the material world. That would be achieved by "one-pointed attention to the object of devotion". The student at that stage "has become oblivious to external stimulation and is brought to the *threshold of consciousness*", the *lowest stage of samadhi* (Malhotra, p. 32, emphasis not included).

Now after the experience of the outer universe is excluded, the inner journey can start, and that journey comprises seven stages all summarized as *samadhi or contemplative consciousness*. It comprises hierarchically ordered seven levels. The two lowest stages are *samprajnata* and *asamprajnata*. In the former consciousness is centred on "reasoning, reflection, joy and ego-sense", in the latter consciousness has "transcended this occupation". Now the two main stages of *samadhi* in the wider sense are entered. One penultimate stage comprises three sub-stages, which are all characterized still by object fixations and therefore named as *samadhi* with a seed (*subija*). The object for *savitarka and nirvitarka* is of "gross matter" while the yogi at the further sub-stage, *savicara,* needs to centre his consciousness only at "subtle substance". Once consciousness needs no object anymore, the ultimate stage is reached, which is the final state of *samadhi* understood in the narrower sense. The beginning stage of this stage is called *nirvicara,* which is described as "devoid of thought" and characterized as "truthbearing wisdom" or "intuitive knowledge". The ultimate stage then is again the transcendence of these two properties and "pure consciousness" is achieved, the *nirbija samadhi*. Patanjali dedicated three sutras to the last *nirbija* stage in which "the seedless stage of mental stillness arises" (1.51). After this ultimate union with the all-pervading cosmic consciousness has been achieved the individual still sees and experiences the world through the mind but without the wrong identifications, being the cause of all sufferings (*sadhanapada sutras*). The difference between samadhi states "with and without a seed" might have been at the root of a controversy following contradictory results regarding its expressions of samadhi in the EEG as will be discussed in the next section.

Bagchi &Wenger (1957) tried to translate the endeavour to reach 'one-pointed attention of devotion' by a "psycho-physiologico-neuroanatomical figure of speech". According to that the yogis attempted

"to use the attention phenomenon of the cortex to merge into and stabilize at a different level the 'indeterminate awareness' of the deep subcortical mechanism, the highest plane of neural integration – the centrencephalon" (p136).

Namely consciousness is indeed not there just to be found, it has to be achieved or created by an "evolutionary process" in the human brain which takes place "through accessory disciplines buttressed by this prolonged, quiet one-pointed meditation and consequent strengthening of the cortical dynamism". "True self-control, knowledge, and happiness as well as freedom from false beliefs and attitudes, liberated lives" (ibidem) would be the expression of this achievement.

An excursion into a *Vedic* philosophical concept has been undertaken in order to provide the psycho-physiologico-neuroanatomical background that Indian meditation practices are based on. In the following section on the early if not "classic" studies of meditation research the EEG results will be at first reported almost exclusively while the autonomous measurements will be reported in a later section. Here it is intended to give a review on the brain processes as far as they are accessible by the crude results the EEG could deliver.

The early studies – is *Samadhi* activating?

Das & Gastaut (1957) gave the first report in 1955 on a conference in Lausanne and that has mostly been the cited date of the paper. They investigated seven yogis of both genders from one and the same yogic community in their laboratory in New Delhi. Electric brain activity was measured for each subject during eight subsequent phases: Beginning stage in cross legged sitting position (lotus or *padmasan*), breathing exercises (pranayama), light meditation, deep meditation, very deep meditation or exstatic, (exstasy or samadhi) and one hour after samadhi, achieved by one exceptional subject (Haridas). For *all* subjects, however, the alpha activity of the beginning stage (sitting in a crosslegged position) was not modified in any way by posture and breathing exercises that followed. The EEG showed:

> "...progressive and very spectacular modifications during the deepest meditations, in those subjects who have the best training:
>
> a) acceleration (1-3 cps) of the alpha rhythm, decrease of the amplitude, and appearance of faster (15, 20, 30 cps) components.
>
> b) A beta rhythm of 18-20 cps in the rolandic areas.
>
> c) A generalized fast activity of small amplitude, which may reach 25-30 cps and sometimes even 40-45 cps.
>
> d) During the samadhi period, the generalized fast rhythms may be of higher amplitude, reaching 30 and 50 microvolts.
>
> e) During and after meditation, the alpha rhythm reappears, often slower and more widely distributed at first (8 and even 7 cps)."

There were no changes of the fast rhythms of high amplitude recorded by the EEG after acoustic, photic, tactile and even nociceptive stimulations applied during the samadhi stage. This insensitivity was accompanied by immobility and palor, symptoms which are known by the Indian tradition being characteristic for samadhi and by psychiatrists interpreted as signs of coma. Furthermore there was no activity recorded by the EMG. The authors thoroughly discussed the possibility of an EMG artefact biasing the EEG results, because those were within the range of the fast rhythms. It could have been the case that the EEG electrodes picked up muscular activity in the scalp. However, the authors excluded such a possibility. Not only the temporal electrodes of the rolandic (= central) areas had detected the fast rhythms but also the electrodes on the vertex (where no muscles exist!) had.

They concluded that yogi meditation and the ecstasy to which it leads represent a state of intense concentration of attention. Furthermore they suggested that this concentration on the object of meditation elicited general cortical stimulation, which was responsible for the insensitivity during *samadhi*. Thereby they declared, they had provided a more parsimonious explanation than others, suggesting local or diffuse inhibition not permitting stimuli to come through to the cortex in such cases.

A few years later in another New Delhi laboratory, Anand, Chhina and Singh (1961) investigated four yogis who belonged to another type of yoga school (*raja*) with a similar design. All four yogis achieved a samadhi-state and with two of them insensitivity to stimulation in the acoustic, visual and tactile modality was replicated. However, the fast rhythms reported by Das & Gastaut earlier were not found in the EEG-records of these subjects: they showed alpha rhythms all along the meditation stages with increased amplitude modulation in *samadhi*. One of these yogis also practiced "pin-pointing consciousness": the ability to concentrate attention on different points of the vault of the skull. The authors, however, did not further discuss this result, and it was not explained what the point in reporting this exercise was. Today this might be interesting for a spotlight theory of attention (Wolfe, 1994).

The studies of Bagchi & Wenger (1957) and Wenger and Bagchi (1961) also rather supported Anand, Chhina & Singh's findings. They investigated yogis from all over the country in different laboratories run by state yoga institutes, and one they visited in his cave in the Himalayas whereto they had lugged up their equipment. They made different physiological investigations on a number of issues, which of meditation was only one. They found insensitivity to high stimulation in the environment with several subjects. One yogi was already during the application of the electrodes completely immobile and without tonus, the EMG showed no activation at all. All subjects showed a clear alpha pattern at the beginning of meditation and increased amplitudes in states of deep meditation. However, none of their 14 subjects achieved a samadhi-state according to subjective assessment. They concluded that meditation leads to a state of deep relaxation of the autonomic nervous system without drowsiness or sleep. They considered three explanations for the insensitivity all having to do with consciousness going somewhere subcortical. It is quoted here:

> "If this non-perception of stimuli is a fact then meditation may represent a twilight-state in which stimulus response reflex probably functions, if it functions at all, in the form of palmar resistance change or EEG blocking, below the cortical level – below the level of undetermined awareness. Or, the prolonged non-perception of such stimuli may be primarily a cortical affair – the overall quiet turbulence or willed meditation-state making ineffective the small ripples caused by extraneous stimuli, with the preservation of subcortical reflex action. …there must be a persistent EEG adaptation phenomenon … as commonly seen in EEG of ordinary persons during continuous endogenous or exogenous stimuli. Or, this non-perception may be an indirect result of a cortico-subcortical tug-of-war with one-pointedness of conscious will finally merging itself and stabilizing itself at a different level of the highest integrating subbcortical neural mechanism associated with "indeterminate" awareness." (p.142).

Anand et al did not bother to explain insensitivity to intense stimulation. They did instead feel necessary to explain the alpha rhythm by autonomous discharge of the reticular activating system. Not insensitivity during alpha rhythms was the problem but alpha rhythms during an unconscious state. These authors took *samadhi* for being a state of *coma* without mentioning it though. However, then the ease to get into such a state and getting out of it again would be the "meditation problem" as Bagchi & Wenger before had called it at the end of their discussion.

Since research in the next 20-30 years showed predominantly alpha rhythms in meditation states the results of the Das & Gastaut study were dismissed as artifactual (Fenwick, 1987) in spite of the authors' thorough discussion of that possibility across half a page. The problem for the reviewers was then that the description of where exactly the electrodes had been attached to the skull was relatively inexact. There was no international standardization scheme of the locations before 1958.

However, beta rhythms were later also found by another French researcher - in a Harvard laboratory (Banquet, 1973) - by comparing meditators of the transcendental meditation technique (TM) with experience from 9 months to 5 years to a matched control sample with relaxation across different phases of meditation or relaxation. (The TM technique involves mainly to take a sitting position and to concentrate with eyes closed on a *sanskrit* word or syllable and turning attention back to the mantra once the mind has drifted away from it.) All 12 meditators had a basic alpha rhythm in the resting record, which became predominant in the beginning stage of the meditation phase. In the actual meditation phase of 30 minutes individual differences were found. While eight meditators had a shift to slower high amplitude rhythms either in the alpha or the even slower *theta* range, four subjects showed a fast and rhythmic beta pattern. Banquet's design recorded precisely the subjective states, i.e. the meditators pushed a button when they entered another mental state during their meditation. It was at the third stage which they later described as "deep meditation or even transcendence" after alpha and theta had been passed through when the four showed fast beta activity at 20 cycles per second (cps). Like Das & Gastaut there were also some rhythms of 40cps belonging actually into the *gamma* range. The fast rhythms had a tendency "to become continuous on a persistent background of slower activity" and spectral analysis showed a rhythmic pattern, which was very different from the fast rhythms produced by the control subjects in relaxation. The chin EMG showed no activity throughout the meditation period in contrast to the resting and post meditation period. The possibility of artefacts due to scalp-muscle activity was practically ruled out by the spectral analytical approach.

The dismissal of Das & Gastaut's study because of EMG artefact is not accepted here for a few reasons.

> The colleagues of Das & Gastaut had only been questioned the fast rhythms only after the immediately following research results had not been found consistent with them. However, the different meanings of the term samadhi may have plaid a role here. The subject Haridas was regarded as an exceptional yogi and might have been the only subject who had achieved the ultimate state of samadhi according to the descriptions by Patanjali, the "seedless" state of complete mental stillness, not onepointedness (subija).

➢ The fast rhythms found by Banquet were clearly not artefactual. The hypothesis about fast rhythms in samadhi should be maintained as long as no more studies on that particular stage of meditation have been conducted. One failure to replicate is by far not sufficient to rule out fast rhythms at this stage.

➢ The artefact theory ignores the course of heart rate synchronous with the rhythms. In general it increased with the beginning of meditation and decreased after it. During deep meditation and samadhi it increased in parallel with the increase of frequency! The samadhi subject for example had an increase of 5bpm during light meditation and another 5bpm during deep meditation and samadhi. After meditation his heart rate decelerated to 70bpm. Before meditation it was 85bpm. The control EMG of the quadriceps in contrast was flat all the time after taking the cross-legged position and that should exclude the hypothesis of cardiosomatic coupling.

➢ All studies were conducted on yogis from different schools. Das & Gastaut had to do with Kriya-Yogis and they have slightly different concepts than Hatha and Raja yogis. They are particularly concerned with the Kundalini theory, assuming that, inherent to all humans, a certain force, "sleeping" at the bottom of the spine was ready to be evoked through certain physical and psychological disciplines.

➢ Experienced genuine yogis are difficult to access as Bagchi and Wenger explained. They emphasised that yogis are not primarily interested in progression of science and to display their abilities is even counter their own philosophy of self-denial and renunciation of self-rewarding attitudes. In Das & Gastaut's case the familiarity between one of the investigators with his subjects from childhood onwards, as explained by the authors, was the best antidote to those abstinent attitudes. Those kriya yogis trusted and were attached to the experimenter and probably wanted to help him by displaying their abilities to full extent. Perhaps only those who are somewhat familiar with the Hindu culture can understand such an argument.

➢ The appreciative, sometimes even devotional style, which the paper was written in, replicated the subjects' affectionate attitude. It is perhaps also this style which raised suspicion about wrong findings assuming that "cool objective" judgement might have gone down with devotion. However, that would be a mistake, on the contrary, every author should write beforehand what interest he pursues with his investigation and a distant writing style does not necessarily reflect objectivity in research attitude at all, or does it? In this case even being on the side of the subjects was even just the right approach. A positive climate is at the beginning of the learning of any meditation novice and the philosophy of meditation demands positive thinking for any creative action. The authors just supported the efforts of the subjects to achieve their results by a postitive attitude

➢ By the same token the subjects of Bagchi & Wenger but particularly of Anand et al. might perhaps not have gone to the highest possible stage in their meditations. In the former case the subjects had made that clear: only the "precincts of samadhi" had been achieved (p.315). The latter authors claimed samadhi stages had been achieved, however, their interpretation of samadhi as an unconscious state and their failure to discuss the pin-pointing exercise of one of the yogis shows that they had an interest in debunking the "hype" surrounding the "problem of meditation". It is highly unlikely that the *raja* yogis would not have known their attitude since such people have a high degree of mind-reading capacity, whether such a thing is based on behavioural indicators or on pure intuition. Hence the claims of these authors that their subjects had achieved samadhi states can at the very least equally be taken with caution as the description of the electrode-positioning in the methods section by Das & Gastaut.

This was the first controversy in research on meditation. By dismissing Das & Gastaut's results as artefactual the picture of meditation as a relaxation technique leading into alpha states in parallel with autonomous indicators of relaxation had emerged. The majority of studies supported indeed this view, but there are exceptions as will be shown in the next section. Before that two other controversies of EEG research on meditation have to be reported. One is about meditation leading to a state similar to sleep, the other on hemispherical specificity of meditation effects.

Meditation and Sleep

The theta trains Banquet found with his meditators were not the first ones.

Earlier research on Japanese priests and their students (Kasamatsu & Hirai, 1966) practising *zazen,* a technique that involves counting the breaths with eyes opened and starting on one again as soon as the meditator is lost in other mental activities. These subjects showed different wave patterns in the EEG at different stages of meditation. Alpha waves do not usually appear in the EEG when the subject's eyes are open (higher frequency beta waves are typical then) and neither do the lower frequency, high amplitude theta waves (5-7 Hz). However, alpha waves of 11-12 Hz appeared with all subjects and tetha trains occurred with those priests who had practiced for about 20 years. Further, there were high correlations between the proficiency ratings given by the masters and the students performance of high amplitude / low frequency EEG patterns. The student's numbers of practising years were not predictive for those patterns.

Theta waves usually indicate deep sleep; however, there are differences between the regular theta pattern appearing in the spectrum, often described as "trains" recorded in meditation and the more irregular pattern in deep sleep. Then, one priest showed no habituation to orienting stimuli (clicks), i.e. he responded to every click as if he had heard it for the first time.

While the dishabituation to clicks has not been replicated with alpha waves either (Becker & Shapiro, 1981), theta-waves have been shown as specific to meditation in a controlled study with western subjects reported by Fenwick (1969) reported in the same author's review (1987). His subjects were meditators using a purely mental mantra-technique similar to TM. These subjects were all quite experienced meditators and asked in a random order to either meditate or to drowse. There was a typical pattern of alpha waves followed by theta trains for the meditation condition. Computer analysis and blind ratings of the EEG records showed reliable differences between drowsiness and the meditative condition.

Also Hebert & Lehmann (1977) reported on theta trains in meditation and Corby, Roth et al (1978) whose results in autonomous variables will be reported later found theta waves with experienced meditators in their EEG more than with control subjects (beginners). Most remarkable was at the time that the meditators showed theta also in their normal consciousness raising the question whether this was an effect of training or of selection. On the other hand expert meditators and the tradition claim that the practice changes normal consciousness and the finding confirms that claim for the time being.

Hemispheric effects?

Fenwick (1987) speculated about an interaction effect of cognition and physiological relaxation, i.e. holistic philosophy and meditation experience at the onset stage of sleep resulting in a right hemispherical view on the world. He mentioned a case study in which a *Zen* master showed normal left hemispherical function in an intelligence test but an entirely right hemispheric approach in dealing with the world in a dynamic interview he conducted with him. It seems that the *Zen* master's communication skills in response to western psychiatric methodology had been heavily tested in that dynamic interview, one may speculate back. He might have responded just with that extreme kindness that can be demonstrated by Asian masters in response to inquisitive behaviour natural to western but not Asian minds. In any case, Pagano & Warrenburg (1983) could not find enough evidence in reviewing the literature to support the hypothesis for a meditation training induced shift from left more linear to right more holistic hemispheric information processing styles.

The Ganzfeld-and-Stabilised-Image Theory of Meditation

Hence, *concentration* is one common element of all meditation techniques. Ornstein (1972) regarded *repetition* as the second and took evidence from the vision research field for the hypothesis that stabilisation of sensory input leads to *turn off* or *blank out* which is the short-term purpose of meditation techniques. He related *satory,* those meditative states that happen for novice meditators in a "split of a second" to the effects of *Stabilised Im*age and *Ganzfeld.*

Stabilizing an image means to abolish the continuous changes of input that normally occur in processes of vision and that is due to the saccade movements of the eye for overall vision and optical *nystagmus* when objects are fixed. Because of these movements, the objects on the retina are kept in constant motion. A theory evolved around the *oculomotoric* particularities according to which normal awareness could only be maintained under such constantly changing input conditions. The reverse would be evidence for absence of awareness when a visual object is kept stable on the retina. Such evidence was provided by Pritchard (1961) with the help of a device that induced this condition: A tiny projector was mounted on a contact lens worn by the subject and independent from the eye movements the image was constantly projected on the retina. The effect was that the image disappeared after a few moments. However, as Ornstein reported in some studies the image tended to reappear periodically, which he ascribed to the slipping of the lens, i.e. to the inconstancy of condition. Ornstein claimed that under extreme constant conditions the image would disappear in a few seconds and never return (p 164). Another research team found alpha waves in the EEG related to the stabilised image (Lehmann, Beeler & Fender, 1967).

The effect of the white wall that the Japanese priests of Kasamatsu & Hirai were gazing at before their brain produced alpha patterns had been investigated in the laboratory already in the fifties by Hochberg, Triebel & Seaman (1951) and by Cohen (1957). A completely patternless visual field is called a *Ganzfeld* (German for whole field). The former authors, quite ingeniously, used halved Ping-Pong balls taped over the eyes of the subjects; the latter used two white completely patternless spheres each of one diameter. The effects were similar as for the stabilised image. Some of the subjects reported after 20 minutes absence of any visual experience and called it "blank-out." They could not say during these blank outs whether they had their eyes open or not. Moreover, they could not control their eye movements. Bursts of alpha wave patterns were associated with the blank-out periods and Cohen found that subjects with high alpha EEGs were more susceptible to the blank-out phenomenon. He suggested that the continuous uniform stimulation of the Ganzfeld resulted in failure to produce any image in the consciousness. This suggested a functional similarity between continuous stimulation and no stimulation at all. The Ganzfeld-blank-out hypothesis was confirmed later by a third author (Ornstein, 1972).

The parallels between the two induced visual situations in the laboratory and concentrative meditation practice were intriguing to Ornstein because in both attempts were made to produce *unchanged sensory input*. In both kinds of situations subjective loss of contact with the external world occurred simultaneous to alpha wave patterns in the EEG (see the studies reported above). It could be argued that the phenomenon of blank-out with the Ganzfeld or disappearance of the stabilised image is specific to the peripheral nervous system since they happened to occur in the visual modality alone. However, Ornstein was convinced that the phenomenon is centrally directed because "the effects of the stabilised image are transferred between the eyes, indicating that the disappearance phenomenon must occur somewhere later in the visual system than in the retina"(p.167). Furthermore, auditory stimulation brought the image back into consciousness.

Autonomous responses and the "Relaxation Response"

As it was known already from the early studies: investigating physiological effects of meditation was difficult because the assessment of bodily signals could interfere with the practice of the yogi-subjects. These difficulties seemed to have changed a great deal when Maharishi Mahesh Yogi started teaching a simple concentrative technique becoming known as Transcendental Meditation (TM) to his mainly western students. TM seemed to have instant beneficial effects on a beginners' mental and physical tensions Maharishi's (= the greatest sage) organisation grew fast and world-wide. It was advised to practice two times a day for 15-20 minutes by sitting in a relaxed posture with closed eyes and repeating mentally a mantra. *Vedic* philosophy on "higher consciousness", which an initiated person could tap into by meditation, was part of an initiation-ritual, performed by the teachers who were trained by Mahesh Yogi. In this context, the personal mantra was given to the adepts and if they carried on practising, they could book advanced courses. In such courses they were introduced into advanced techniques called "siddhi-techniques". A *siddhi* in Sanskrit means something like extra sensory perception which could be achieved as a side effect to spiritual advancement, as Patanjali had mentioned in the *vibhutipada sutras* (Malhotra, 2001). However, the use of the term was no more than a promotion skill, the advancement to "siddha" status (practitioners of the siddhi-technique) had little to do with spiritual advancement – it was a sign that someone continued with his practice though. TM-*Siddhas* practice a set of *yoga asanas* (positions) before they start their meditation, which is in general the usual combination meditators of the Hindu tradition are advised to practice.

That is because other than in the mainstream religions here the interactive relationship of body, mind, and spirit were thoroughly reflected instead of being rejected as for example in the Christian tradition (*manicheism)*. Yoga exercises markedly enhance the effect of meditation and one does not wonder that forms of yoga and pranayama (sets of breathing techniques) have recently been "baptised" by the Roman Catholic Church as long before had been *zen*. So, it was no wonder when Wallace (1970), a young TM practitioner publishing the first study on TM before, during and after meditation practice, praised the ease and readiness of students to meditate, and the effortlessness of recruitment for research purpose as a consequence.

Also because of the instant effects on beginners, TM was a very user-friendly technique for researchers too. They could themselves learn to practice meditation and find out about the possibility of transcendental experience without much commitment (a fee had to be paid for the initiation rite and courses were also held on a fee basis). They could also work together with the organisation and get subjects for their laboratory. The consequence was that a body of research on meditators of the beginner stage was growing fast during the seventies, the organisation could back up their advertising with this research body which, however, was not without flaws, as a controversy during the eighties made obvious to the public (see below).

Wallace (1970) found

> reductions of oxygen consumption by 20%,

> of heart rate by 5 bpm and a

> marked increase of galvanic skin-resistance GSR. There was an

> *alpha* wave pattern in the EEG with a few subjects showing a

> short *theta* train.

All data were assessed within an own-control design, i.e. compared to the subject's own baseline period of 5 minutes before meditation, which is the usual procedure in the tradition of psychophysical research since the 19th century. All changes were regarded as being different from sleep or comparable techniques like autosuggestion or hypnosis and clinical application was suggested because of its reduced metabolic state eliciting effects .

This first study contained the major parameters for what was later termed the *relaxation response* (Wallace & Benson, 1972) with the addition of

> decreased concentration of blood lactate and

> stabilised bloodflow to the forearm muscles.

The *relaxation response* was summarized then as a set of *integrated physiological changes*: namely decreased heart rate and oxygen consumption, arterial blood pressure and respiratory rate. A more recent review (Jevening, Wallace & Beidebach, 1992) described the effects of transcendental meditation as an "integrated response with peripheral circulatory and metabolic changes subserving increased central nervous activity". He and his collaborators namely found increased cardiac output and "probable" cerebral bloodflow during meditation (Jevning, Wilson et al, 1978) which could be physiological correlates of alertness, often reported along with feelings of deep relaxation in subjective reports.

That response was elicited "when a subject assumed a relaxed position in a quiet environment, closes his or her eyes, engages in a repetitive mental action, and passively ignores distracting thoughts" (Hoffman, Benson et al., 1981). The response was elicited by individuals who practised "techniques that have existed for centuries, usually within a religious context" (Benson & Friedman, 1985, p. 725). According to the authors it had been early acknowledged that the response could also be achieved by the use of secular techniques like progressive muscle relaxation, autogenic training and hypnosis before entering the hypnotic (unconscious) state. Four elements were commonly included by the techniques: "a repetitive word, sound or prayer, the adoption of a passive attitude, decreased muscle tonus and a quiet environment" (ibidem).

The relaxation response was usually regarded as the homologue to the *tropotrophic* response, another pattern found by the Swiss physiologist Hess (1949, translation 1957) in response to hypothalamic stimulation of the cat's brain. The response comprises all those functions that serve the organism to recover from strain and to conserve energy, hence triggers nutritive and relaxed behaviour. While the defensive response followed posterior stimulation, the *tropotrophic* response was elicited by stimulation of *anterior* structures[6]. Therefore, it was also regarded as the counterpart to Cannon's fight or flight response (Benson & Friedman, 1985).

During the seventies the TM-enthused researchers quite successfully put the suggestions made by Wallace for clinical application of TM into practice. Hypertension was the first successfully treated condition of sympathetic hyperactivation next to drug- and alcohol abuse (Shafii, Lavely et al. 1975, 1976). Particularly the effects of hypertension have been confirmed several times (e.g. Benson & Wallace, 1972; Blackwell, Hanenson et al., 1976). Holmes (1985) listed these results, among other conditions, at the beginning of his revised critical review, which had been published for the first time in the American Psychologist in 1984, obviously with the intention to debunk meditation research as the emperors new clothes. The publication elicited a debate in the same journal between him and some critics. On the one hand, this article had some merit in its thorough methodological analysis and therefore giving meditation research new impulses (West, Shapiro, both 1985). On the other hand it was probably unique in its aggressive polemic style against a successful method of clinical treatment and obviously because of great dislike of the "whole [transcendental] package" (Holmes, 1985) as he called it in a response to a critic. Besides, he was accused for distortions and misrepresentations, which he denied unconvincingly, as will be shown now.

---

[6] Hess regarded the dichotomic structure of the nervous system reflected in the anterior and posterior functional division of the hypothalamus (posterior part rules *ergotrophic*, active behaviour) which today is regarded as "zu allgemein" overgeneralized, Jaenig, 1994, p. 368).

Holmes' (1984, 1987) Critical Review - critically revisited

This section serves two purposes. The main purpose is to review the literature on meditation, in particular those studies that investigated effects of meditation on stressor-responses. Since the meditation research is not possible to be reviewed without including the harsh criticism of Holmes, these are included. However, Holmes will be reviewed critically too by looking at his "reviewing technique" and by checking his claims against reality, i.e. the papers he criticised.

No chances for no-control group designs

Holmes reviewed the literature by dismissing those studies without control-groups: *case studies* like the early studies reported above and those that used an *own-control* design like Wallace (1970). A within-subject control condition has always been to date the acknowledged psychophysical research method to achieve general results on changes the organism undergoes in response to an external or internal stimulus. The case studies allegedly delivered hypotheses, but could not be taken as "empirical tests of effects of meditation" because there had been no control subjects. He considered a between-subject control condition as an absolute must for scientific clinical research in order to demonstrate *"whether or not meditation is more effective than other arousal-reducing strategies such as simply resting"* (e.g. Holmes, 1987, p.83, emphasis included).

TM versus "Simple Resting" - activation during treatment

After this "procrustean" procedure, he reviewed the remaining research in two categories: those controlled studies investigating changes during treatment and those including laboratory stressors. The latter category is being dealt with in the next section.

For the former category he displayed the results of 23 studies in columns of the physiological variables heart rate, electrodermal activity (EDA), respiration, blood pressure, EMG and "others" (neuroendocrinological, temperature, bloodflow). The main point was, to put the activation reducing effects to the sitting position in which the technique is being practised rather than to the meditation process. In theoretical terms he argued with somatic coupling against central nervous steering of activation reduction as the consciousness oriented meditation researchers had done. The table indicating differences between meditators and resters showed overwhelmingly no differences. In four studies meditators showed reliably higher HR than controls during meditation, one study had meditators having lower EDA attributed to higher initial values and therefore to regression to the mean. One study also showed reliably higher respiration rate for meditators. In biomedical variables, some studies showed reliably higher, some reliably lower indicators of activation for meditators.

Substantial objections and Holmes placebo-control group

The author of this thesis has critically looked at some studies.

Firstly: Michaels, Huber & Cann (1976) compared 12 meditators to 18 (or 9, both statements were reported) resting subjects for blood lactate and catecholamine-concentration and found no reliable differences. The control condition was defined as "sitting quietly" by the authors. Holmes himself had conducted a study with equal numbers of meditators and subjects who were "simply resting" and found no differences in activation reducing effects (HR, EDA, Blood Pressure) during treatment (Holmes *et al*, 1983). Secondly: One of those studies showing allegedly reliable HR differences between resting and meditating was Goleman & Schwartz (1976), a study including also a stressor sequence as will be discussed later. Holmes claimed that in this study *meditating* subjects …evidenced greater increases in heart rate than did the resting subjects…" (p. 86, emphasis excluded). This study had a very complex design structure and even by the crudest method of simplification, this sentence is not true.

For a start, there were no "resting" subjects at all as controls! There were 30 "experienced" meditators of the siddhi technique and 30 interested beginners of TM. Both groups (named as "meditators and controls") were randomly allocated to three conditions: expert meditation and beginner meditation with open eyes and closed eyes. The idea was, secondly, to look for *trait* effects (long term vs short term) and *state* effects of meditation within the control-beginner group (closed vs open eyes). The trait effects, however, by far outscored the state effects and the data were presented mainly for groups *across* the three conditions. Hence, there was no such effect as "more increase of HR in meditating subjects." There was one effect differentiating experienced meditators against absolute beginners after stressor impact and that was presented as the main result of this study, which will be dealt with later again in this thesis. Since comparisons during treatment were made in this section, Holmes should have mentioned this effect: 'all subjects across all three conditions exhibited HR decelerations but control-beginners decelerated reliably more than experienced meditators'.

This is interesting for the trait hypothesis and not astonishing at least for an experienced meditator. Someone who has meditated at least for a year in an advanced technique is very likely to be more alert in any sitting position as long as he does something that prevents him from falling asleep. They were asked not to use their own mantra. Conversely, normal, i.e. non-anxious subjects, completely novice to meditation, will have no difficulty to relax in any of these conditions and probably even 'doze off' in the eyes closed resting position.

Shapiro (1985) questioned that the simple resting condition of Holmes own study had been an appropriate placebo control condition. He argued, the subjects may have been using techniques for autosuggestion like "this is the time just to relax" or one may have chosen to focus at one's own breath. Benson & Friedman (1985) pointed at a similar flaw in Holmes evidence. He had used three studies where the resting condition had explicitly involved relaxation techniques, two of them progressive relaxation. The latter claim he admitted and regretted "as one error", the former he denied because the subjects had been only advised *once* for the experiment to "reduce autonomic functioning, relax as much as possible or ignore and render neutral all external stimuli" (Holmes, 1985, p. 730). "In another [study] they were 'simply given a word and told to *meditate* with it'"(ibidem, emphasis excluded). Holmes insisted that in both cases, no other training had been given and therefore Benson & Friedman's argument allegedly was unsubstantiated. Holmes has to be contradicted here. In the second case the subjects were using even a non-cultic mantra meditation technique for the first time and the result only shows the efficiency of that kind of technique. In the first case, the concentration task seemed to be even more complex.

The three research teams knew that simple resting is difficult and therefore they had given their mental relaxation devices. The individual will mentally do something structured in order to relax when he is tense (counting sheep is common antidote to failure to sleep in the German culture) or just fall asleep as we do when we are tired enough. Therefore it is also no wonder that in one of those experiments, which were meant to prove that meditators showed no lower activation in HR and EEG than resting subjects (Holmes 1987, Table 1, p.87), 13 out of 16 subjects were reported to be asleep. This was pointed out by Benson & Friedman (1985) in their rebuttal (among lots of other critical points).

Meditation techniques are designed as concentrative tasks because they aim to make the meditator "to go into zero" (També, 1982, 3, p.5) without falling unconscious. The *zen* master's stick has become famous he uses to hit a student on his back as soon as he gets drowsy or falls asleep. Only advanced meditators can just sit and do nothing than being awake as the EEG studies quoted above have shown. Studies of such advanced meditators with complete physiological profiles are not available yet. That kind of basic research is missing as West (1987) remarked.

Meditation versus therapy and high intensity stimulation - Holmes post-hoc hypotheses: control of autonomic arousal

Holmes put the following hypothesis in front of this part of his review:

> "Subjects who practice meditation are better able to *control* their arousal in threatening situations than are subjects who do not practice meditation"… "because it was widely believed that meditation will facilitate the control of arousal in threatening situations (p. 91, emphasis not included). "

Further, the ability to control activation elicited by a threatening situation would show whether there are differences in the processes involved in resting and meditating. In other words, results from such experiments could give evidence for centrally mediated processes involved in meditation. These are interesting questions, however, he would have to put them in front of a design of his own. The hypotheses of the investigators he reviewed were slightly different, as will be shown. Further, there is a lot "widely believed" about foreign customs, practices, and peoples. Germans who have never lived in London for example tend to believe that London is a rainy and foggy town. That is because of another, fictional Holmes, famous for his detective skills performed and documented in 19th century London, when the gas lanterns scattered across London caused smog everywhere in the city. Germans are still prejudiced about the London climate probably because of Sir Conan Doyle's novels as it is suggested by today's Londoners.

Similarly, people in Kansas, where David Holmes was teaching at the University, might have read in their tabloids about the astonishing abilities of highly advanced meditators namely yogis to control their autonomic nervous system and thereby may have misjudged the purpose of meditation training taken up by a western seeker. That purpose would hardly have been to acquire the ability to control activation in a threatening situation or developing bizarre abilities as described in those case studies (see Ornstein, 1972 for references). Such abilities are not aims commonly pursued even by advanced meditators.

Moreover meditators with such ambitions would certainly not expect progress in a period of time suitable for short-term laboratory investigation.

Anyway, since it has been discovered through biofeedback research that the autonomy of the autonomous nervous system is a myth, western researchers are not impressed anymore by those Indian masters of Yoga. Even rats can be conditioned to vary their skin temperature in the ears although that would not impress a yogi pursuing such abilites. He only wants to show that man can indeed gain control over his own animal functions by power of his mind. That is because the yogi has a dualistic view on the mind body relationship. He would rather encourage the researcher to practice biofeedback techniques on himself in order to get in touch with his own organism. [7] Control over body and mind is indeed a long-term target of *yogic* practice, but not in order to impress but to achieve spiritual aims, which, for some reason, are not understood by most western psychologists, it seems. The TM organisation had propagated TM to help people with mental and physical tensions (e.g. Wallace, 1970). They certainly had not advertised with learning the capacity to control their heart rate. They were not teaching biofeedback techniques, were they!

Then: If someone has achieved such an extraordinary ability to control arousal, what would it be good for in a threatening situation? Would it not depend on the nature of the threat? Anyway, would not preparing for action be the right purpose of such control ability instead of going into some state of deep meditation as indicated by the EEG with alpha waves pattern and patches of theta trains. Only a fool would advise such a response to a real threat. However, in a simulated situation as a laboratory experiment that would be something interesting to test advanced yogis for, provided they would be interested in showing their abilities. Nevertheless, for meditation beginners, even more advanced TM-siddhas, a preparation for action would be nothing to worry about, or would it?

The four studies: Holmes review and what they really reported

After putting post-hoc the "widely believed" arousal-control-hypothesis to the test, the four studies, naturally, failed to confirm. The problem with Holmes review technique is that he reduced every study to the response to the question: Is there more reduction of activation than for relaxation and/or therapeutic interventions? There was no experiment showing meditators less activated than relaxation controls. Holmes stressed that some studies even showed meditators being reliably more activated than controls (Puente & Beiman, 1980; Lehrer, Schoickett *et al.*, 1980 and Goleman & Schwartz, 1976). According to his arousal-control hypothesis, the meditators were less in control of their activation than the subjects were of the competing methods. Let us look at the studies a bit more in detail.

Goleman & Schwartz, 1976: This study was widely regarded as having produced evidence for meditators exhibiting faster recovery times from stressor impact than beginners and was (and *is*) being used by TM instructors to explain the beneficial effects of TM. Holmes simply ignored the main results as will be shown. (Apart from that he ignored Orme-Johnson's controlled study (1973) on recovery from stressor-impact.)

The authors of this study compared rather experienced TM meditators of the siddhi technique (1-2 years) to beginner meditators without previous experience but with an

---

[7] Biofeedback practices are also part of the rich arsenal of yoga techniques as is progressive muscle relaxation.

interest in learning meditation. These two groups were randomly assigned to one meditation condition and to two relaxation conditions and compared in their anticipation of and response to a film accident. Personality and anxiety questionnaire data were also taken. It was predicted that

a) The meditation condition would display less autonomic arousal and experience less subjective anxiety in response to the film stressor than subjects in the relaxation condition and

b) Experienced meditators would have response patterns and personality traits more consistent with the expected meditation state effects" (p. 457).

The results were structured according to four periods of physiological measurement: resting baseline, treatment period, anticipation period, stressor impact the second of which has been reported in the previous paragraph. There were more effects due to trait than to state or, put another way, more between group than treatment effects: Experienced meditators across conditions were reliably more sympathetically activated, indicated by HR and frequency of skin conductance responses, during one minute of anticipating the film accidents.

During impact of all three film-accidents, both groups had increased activation levels in both parameters but there was a group difference in the average mean of the three post impact recovery periods for both HR and spontaneous skin conductance response (SSCR). The experienced meditators showed a deeper recovery composite mean from the three stressor-impacts than the controls, again regardless of treatment-condition. In order to control for regression to the mean, suggested by the higher anticipatory levels of the meditators, sub-samples of the groups were matched on the pre-stimulus values and analysed. The between group effects remained in both parameters hence suggesting faster recovery on average for all three accident-stimuli.

There was one state effect (Group X Condition): The control- beginner subjects who had meditated on a mantra, performed worst at recovery from stressor impact as a composite while those experienced meditators who meditated (by not using their personal mantra!) recovered best. However, the SSCR data had shown different picture at least in recovery from the first film accident: the meditating control beginners recovered reliably faster from that, but this pattern was not maintained with repetition.

The authors discussed their results by putting all the physiological and psychometric data together to the following concept: The anticipatory activation of the experienced meditators in SCL and HR was interpreted as a defensive response "…that combines both a set to respond and a sensitisation to incipient stimuli"(p 465). By referring to Lazarus & Averill (1972) they stressed "that in a threatening situation anxiety and accompanying physiological activation is adaptive insofar as it prepares the organism for vigilance in order to facilitate appropriate coping reactions" (ibidem). The anticipatory defensive response would become only maladaptive when it failed to habituate. Therefore an adaptive reaction to a passive coping task would be "principally in terms of recovery not in terms of coping actions while under stress" (ibidem). Since the recovery of the experienced meditators was genuine and not regression to the mean as evidenced by comparisons based on pre-stimulus baseline matched samples, they concluded, that long term meditation practice therefore had facilitated adaptive stress responses. The recovery hypothesis was also backed by the results in anxiety and related measures. The meditators had reliably lower anxiety and neuroticism scores than the control beginners and that will be reported in the appropriate section.

Holmes (1984) found worth while reporting only that

❖ the meditators' group had been more activated throughout the experimental session, thereby including the deceleration during treatment (discussed here under heading Substantial Objections) and unreliable, tonic differences;

❖ the meditators' group exhibited more anticipatory activation than control beginners in skin conductance response frequency.

❖ The recovery issue he treated as follows (in both versions, 1985, 1987 p. 94): He picked exclusively the terms "defensive response" and "increased vigilance" from the discussion and labelled it as an "interesting speculation" without any evidence. Namely, the meditators recovered only to their own elevated pre-stimulus baseline in SCL. According to Holmes, they ought to have had recovered to the initial lower baselines of the control beginners. Then, the authors allegedly only "argued" that there was no regression to the mean. The pre-stimulus matched samples (of appropriate sizes) in both variables Holmes had simply not mentioned. This result implied that also meditators with *lower* pre-stimulus baselines had recovered faster from the film-accidents too. Did Holmes perhaps not know what a baseline matched sample is?

For the author of this thesis it is difficult to understand this denial of statistical evidence, because the t-statistics had been given in all matched sample cases and if he found that was not enough he should have pointed that out. He could also have asked the authors for information that is more elaborate, as it is the custom in such case.

Let us return to the discussion of Goleman & Schwartz (1976). There the authors had appreciated cognitive restructuring work on the appraisal of threat but gave the work on recovery from stress an equal importance with reference to studies on habituation. The stressor response with a fast recovery for the meditators represented indeed the opposite of a response of highly anxious persons.

The authors also discussed the possibility of lifestyle variables like vegetarianism, less stimulans intake etc., and self-selection contributing to the favourable trait result for the experienced meditators. They argued that the state (treatment) effects of meditation (at least in SSCR) would support some contribution of the variable meditation. Therefore, they suggested long-term longitudinal studies [8].

Holmes also treated the other studies with obvious bias.

Puente & Beiman, 1980: This study used a sample of 60 self-referred anxious volunteers and allocated them randomly to four conditions: a) cognitive behavioural therapy (CBT) progressive muscle relaxation (PMR), TM and waiting-list-control (WL). There were seven treatment sessions (90 min) distributed over 4 weeks and measurement

---

[8] However, the author of this thesis has doubts that a longterm study isolating a meditation–technique would be difficult to conduct. That is because meditation practice in itself, in the long run, produces a change of lifestyle (e.g. vegetarianism).

of heart rate and subjective response to aversive slides was taken one each before and after this whole period. CBT and PMR habituated from about 2 bpm in the first to less than 0.4 in the second session while TM and WL rather sensitised from 1.4 bpm and 0.9 bpm to 1.8 bpm respectively 1.2 bpm. These differences were reliable between the groups. It was not presented that the self-relaxation condition also had a powerful therapeutic component. However, already in the abstract Puente & Beiman suggested to interpret these differences "as resulting from therapeutic suggestion and positively reinforced client progress "(p.291). The CBT and PMR group had been told in each of the seven sessions that the treatment would promote client control over physiological arousal. This suggestion was mentioned in the TM condition only once and obviously not at all in the WL condition. Furthermore, CBT and PMR therapists "consistently reinforced client reports of extra session progress on tension-related problems. The TM instructor did not interact with participants in such a way as to determine whether therapeutic progress was taking place" (ibidem, p.295). Indeed the study could not provide evidence for the "reputed psychotherap-eutic benefits of TM" (ibidem) as the authors concluded and the whole idea of the study obviously was to show superiority of behaviourist psychotherapy over TM at least in the short-term. Nevertheless, Holmes obviously had "forgotten" to report anything of that clinically interesting sophisticated detail, because he probably wanted to make PMR look superior too. He presented the study as another example of TM failing to prove arousal control in a threatening situation in competition with therapy and self-relaxation.

Lehrer, Schoickett, Woolfolk & Carrington, 1980: 36 subjects had been randomly selected for PMR and a clinical version of TM, i.e. a mantra meditation without cultic aspects, a secularised version called clinically standardised meditation (CSM) designed by the latter author. After a treatment period of five to six weeks, the subjects underwent one physiological experiment with 5 tones of 100 dB and 500 Hz frequency as stressor-stimuli and HR, SCL as physiological measures and questionnaire anxiety measures. There were reliable initial and pre-stimulus resting differences between meditation and relaxation group, the meditators being higher by 13 bpm. There had been no differences in the accelerative response to the tones and the meditators decelerated more in recovery. The effect remained highly significant (p<0.001) by analysing the data with the pre-stimulus levels as covariates. Therefore, the differences in recovery needed not to be attributed to the initial differences. The fast recovery hypothesis found some support in the frontal EEG that showed in all post-stimulus windows of 2.5 sec overall more alpha waves for the meditators. These differences were marginally reliable after the penultimate tone and reliable after the last tone.

The authors interpreted the initial resting (5 min.) and pre-tone differences as "anticipatory effects" thereby referring to Goleman & Schwartz (1976). The meditators had produced an "anticipatory coping response" because they had shown higher heart rate only in the pre-stimulus period. However, this interpretation cannot be agreed with. There was hardly a difference between initial resting period and pre-tone period (p=0.9!). It looked rather like tonic differences between relaxation and meditation group in spite of random group allocation. There was yet another problem: only seven meditators and six relaxers and eleven control subjects had taken part in this experiment. Almost 50% had dropped out during treatment.

Holmes neither made mention of the quite convincing evidence for greater recovery in heart rate nor did he mention the partially concomitant EEG results. Instead he focussed on the higher activation during anticipation in HR-forearm and frontalis- and forearm EMG and did not mention the striking initial differences in heart rate, the actual snag in the report of this study, nor the coping response hypothesis. Interestingly, Holmes (1984, 1987) did not include at all the following study of the previous authors in any edition of his review.

Lehrer, Woolfolk *et al.*, (1983) partially intended to confirm the Goleman & Schwartz (1976) findings by comparing CSM and PMR (again only by one physiological experiment) in response to five loud tones (100dB) and additionally to that accident- film. Only anxious subjects were taken this time as volunteers because the high drop-out rate of the earlier study was attributed to lack of treatment motivation. The drop-out rate was far less dramatic this time and the study confirmed significant between group difference in recovery heart rate deceleration (difference between pre- and post-stimulus minimum heart rate) after each of the loud tones. There were no between group differences in heart rate (and SCL) during resting or stimulation by tones or film accidents.

There were group differences in forearm and frontalis-EMG: The latter differentiated between treatment groups and control group during the tones. Waiting-list-controls increased muscle activity reliably more than meditation and relaxation group during and after impact, indicating higher stress responses. The relaxation group exhibited reliably less activity in the forearm EMG during the film than meditation and control group. There were no differences in SCL found anywhere. The questionnaire data of this study are treated in the section on subjective measurements below.

Conclusions for the task

A *passive* concentrative technique like TM does not reduce anticipatory activation, rather the effect seems to be enhancing: Two of the studies have given some evidence for more physiological activation in anticipation of high intensity stressors. On the other hand those studies also reported faster recovery of meditators from stressor impact. The meditators' experience ranged from five weeks to two years.

Relaxation response model versus proficiency model

Holmes left out also the following prominent particularly innovative study from the seventies. It questioned the relaxation response model of meditation suggesting the *proficiency model* instead (Corby, Roth *et al.*, 1978). It was claimed that at the beginner's stage of meditation a state of relaxation is predominant but that for experienced meditators, like yogis for example, meditation is a highly active process that would be expressed in higher physiological activation during meditation. They referred to Das & Gastaut (1955) who had those fast frequencies occurring in *samadhi* reported by the highly trained yogis, but which had been regarded as artifactual by the reviewers (see previous section on EEG).

Wenger & Bhagchi (1961) had investigated the meditation of "older yogis" and yoga students and found different patterns of activation in three measurements taken on three consecutive days. The Yogis had faster heart rate (5 bpm), higher systolic blood pressure (20mmHg) and higher palmar skin conductance than the students. Respiratory rates were slightly lower for the yogis as were finger temperatures. The authors therefore interpreted the differences as suggesting that "for these yogis the process [of meditation] is an active one, not a passive, relaxed contemplation" (p.315).

Corby, Roth *et al* (1978) studied another concentrative meditation technique than TM, namely *tantric meditation,* within and between three subject groups. Two groups of meditators with different lengths of experience: *trainees* with 2.1 years and daily practice of 3.4 hours on average and *experts* with 4.4 years of practice and daily meditation practice of 3.4 hours. Both trainees and experts were recruited from a monastic style institute that demanded considerable ethical commitment from its students. A third group was a beginner group of college students with no experience at all who were told to meditate on a mantra of their own choice. The average age of each group was below 26 years.

Each subject received three 20-minute-tone sequences as background to their practice with two kinds of tones to elicit cortical potentials for the EEG. Those sequences also included four white noise stimuli of 70dB to elicit an orienting response. The subjects had all to go through three conditions each seemingly of 20 minutes duration. One resting period of normal consciousness, one period of giving attention to their own breathing named as *withdrawal* phase and one of actual meditation: repeating a two syllable personal mantra given by their teachers in phase with the breathing. The control-beginner group chose their own word.

The other discriminative variable in Corby, Roth *et al.*'s approach is "strength of concentration" within the subcategory "concentrative techniques". The technique used in this study comes from the *tantric* tradition involving "intense concentration of attention". Since the technique we will employ for our study is also a *tantric* technique the authors' explanation of the term is quoted here:

> "The tantric tradition has ancient roots that may antedate *yoga,* but it has now been incorporated into the devotional tradition in *yoga.* The *tantric* tradition emphasises that all the energies of the organism are potentially capable of transformation into the spiritual energy of union with the object of devotion. It is probable that the *kriya* meditators studied by Das & Gastaut (1955) were from the *tantric* tradition since their techniques utilised *tantric* concepts of *kundalini* (spinal energy source) and *chakras* (spinal energy sites) (p. 572)."

The authors' hypothesis of more sympathetic activation in meditation with years of practice was impressively confirmed in all the variables.

Conditions, Skin conductance: There were reliable differences between meditators and control-beginners in skin conductance level in the withdrawal and meditation phase, the meditators being higher as a group, but the trainees being (insignificantly) higher than experts. All meditators reliably increased their levels relative to controls as they went from normal consciousness into meditation. However, interestingly the experts reduced SCL like the controls during withdrawal, and became activated only while meditating. The trainees were activated at the withdrawal stage relative to the normal consciousness-resting phase already and remained at the same heightened level during meditation. SSRR indicated even stronger between group differences. These three findings suggested that the experts had control over their meditative and withdrawal state and the trainees not. The meditators showed higher frequencies of SC responses in withdrawal and meditation than controls. The difference was highest in the meditation phase between experts and controls.

There were no differences reported for heart rate, however, the experts exhibited a linear increase from normal to meditative state of 2.4 bpm. The changes of controls and trainees were below 1 bpm.

Orienting Response HR: there were clear and reliable differences between the meditators and controls in orienting to the white noise stimuli in all three conditions. Both groups had bi-phasic responses in normal resting consciousness, but there was a difference in shape: both groups exhibited the typical primary acceleration to the stimulus and meditators then showed the expected deceleration. The controls in this phase had another acceleration. However, more importantly, in the withdrawal condition the control beginners exhibited a clear deceleration (minimum 1.5 bpm) right from stimulus onset while the meditators equally clearly accelerated (peak 3 bpm). During the meditation phase the meditators accelerated again though less (peak 2 bpm) in response to the stimulus. In this phase, the control beginners showed the typical biphasic response of orienting. SCL: There were insignificant differences with the meditators showing less SSCR in all conditions.

EEG: The meditators increased their alpha power with meditation more than the controls but not reliably: Meditators showed reliably more theta power overall than the controls. The difference between experts and controls for the single conditions was reliable only in normal consciousness though. Hence, the meditators in spite of being more activated physiologically than the control beginners showed no signs of activation in their EEG, moreover they were cortically more deactivated.

This study was unique in using western practitioners, varying in experience of a meditation technique that required more practice time (one hour) and more active concentration, namely attention to breathing, and then mantra focussing along with the breath. The authors' proficiency hypothesis thus was confirmed by their own study because all the results showed a linear increase of sympathetic activation with experience, reversely, a negative relationship of relaxation with experience.

It seems appropriate to reconsider the result from the Goleman & Schwartz study with regard to the decreased deceleration during treatment and the anticipatory activation to the impending film accidents. They were all proficient meditators of the siddhi technique and thus been given more concentration task. In the light of Corby, Roth *et al* (1978) study the vigilance hypothesis, starkly refuted by Holmes, becomes even more likely: As Corby *et al.* speculated,

> "meditative techniques in general permit access to a state of consciousness in the borderline between sleep and wakefulness. Those techniques that employ longer meditation…would be expected to be accompanied by greater physiological activation than shorter meditation techniques (p. 577)."

Since the siddhas (TM meditators using siddhi technique) were asked to meditate one hour at a time, they do fall into the category of longer meditation practice. The authors then suggested that the activation may reflect *progressive conditioning* as subjects attempt to meditate without falling asleep. This would apply to the treatment phase of the Goleman &

Schwartz study, where the meditators decelerated their heart rate less than the control beginners.

In terms of proficiency as the main differentiating factor between meditation practices also Holmes study on resting versus TM deserves the criticism made by Shapiro (1985). He had used a mixture of TM beginners and siddhas and found meditators even more activated during meditation.

Summary (Critical View on a Critical Review)

Holmes (1984, 1987) made some valid points in objecting to

➢ Own control designs in clinical research:

➢ Ignoring initial differences for physiological analysis

➢ Possible bias of self selection in effects on meditation

It cannot be agreed with his reviewing technique, excluding relevant research through

➢ 4.1 Questionable criteria: Between-subject differences across competing conditions are necessary to evaluate a method's efficiency relative to the aims of the investigation. However, one has to regard the within-subjects changes as most important for evaluation of the effects of a stimulus as it has always been in psychophysical research tradition. By excluding case studies and own control design based research Holmes could circumvent for example the intriguing within-subject changes found in the EEG measures by Banquet. Cutting off the origins of research into meditation alone by misusing an empiricist argument hinted at a negative bias against the whole research area.

➢ 4.2 Completely unknown criteria: Most importantly he did not include the innovative study of Corby, Roth *et al* (1978) which would have given him the opportunity to think about the bi-directional issue of proficiency. He repeatedly addressed this issue as a unidirectional one assuming that the capacity to relax would increase with experience.

➢ Distorting and misrepresenting many other results as has been shown.

➢ Using non-cultic meditation techniques similar to clinically standardized meditation as "mock-meditations" for control groups *(this will be further substantiated in the paragraphs discussing Smith's research on anxiety in the following section.).*

1.7.3. Personality, Anxiety, Mood and Stress Management

Cognitive measures like mood and trait and state anxiety can show long term effects of stress management and are therefore to be included in a study of this type. Also personality scores have occasionally been found to show effects.

Extraversion

According to Delmonte's review (1987) several studies employing TM as a technique have reported differences in Extraversion. Self selected meditators scored lower on Extraversion than controls (e.g. West, 1980). Some studies showed TM meditators becoming more extravert with continued practice, others not.

Anxiety, State and Trait

Based on factor analysing questionnaire data of psychiatric patients, anxiety has been separated into cognitive and somatic aspects (Delmonte, 1987 for reference). Cognitive anxiety is measured by paper-pencil-tests; somatic anxiety by degree of sympathetic activation dissociated from exercise. Anticipatory activation of a threatening stimulus is usually regarded as somatic anxiety. While Benson, Beary et al (1974) claimed that the relaxation response generally works on both aspects of anxiety, Davidson & Schwartz (1976) proposed that stress management methods work on those aspects which they employ. Thus, a somatic method like PMR would work on somatic anxiety, meditation as a cognitive method would affect cognitive anxiety. That theory has been given only weak evidence by research (Schwartz, Davidson et al 1978).

The studies of Goleman & Schwartz (1976) and Lehrer et al. (1980, 1983) showed meditation as a good means to reduce state anxiety. The earlier study showed significant differences between the meditators and control beginners before entering the laboratory and after the film-accident (see previous section). They also scored reliably lower on trait anxiety and neuroticism (EPQ), which is correlated with trait anxiety. This is an interesting result because in many studies (e.g. West 1980) prospective meditators had been found being more trait-anxious than the general population. Since both groups in this study were self-selected the hypothesis could be supported that meditation reduces both state and trait anxiety. However, those individuals who regularly drop out from laboratory studies play an important role here. Those with lower levels might continue and the more anxious persons might drop out.

Lehrer, Schoickett et al. (1980) found significant decrements only when the treatment groups were combined and compared to the waiting list controls. The decrements in the meditation group were relatively larger. In their second study (1983) reliable differences were found for trait anxiety in both meditation and PMR group after four months of treatment with greater changes in the PMR group, but no significant changes were found for state anxiety. The subjects had to anticipate a stress experiment only in the post treatment, which explained this result. The relaxation group nevertheless showed a "borderline significant decrease" and the control group a borderline significant increase of state anxiety scores. There is a bulk of studies with randomised and pre-post design structure that proved relaxation and other competing procedures like biofeedback, exercise and "credible control procedures" (Delmonte, 1987, p.122) being equal in improving state anxiety levels. Some studies resulted in meditation being superior to competing methods like eyes-closed-rest-practice or counselling (Dillbeck, 1977; Linden, 1973). Some studies also found differences between meditators and relaxers in the evaluation of their meditative or relaxed states (Morse, Martin *et al.* 1977 and Gilbert, Parker *et al.*, 1978). Curtis & Wessberg, (1975/76) found meditators had more positive mood after meditation than controls after relaxation.

Thus, both meditation and progressive muscle relaxation seem to reduce state anxiety. Delmonte concluded in his review that meditation and other treatments as mentioned above have equally reliable effects on state and trait anxiety with exception of progressive muscle relaxation. However, both Lehrer *et al.* studies proved effects for both PMR and meditation, the later study even showed greater effects for PMR (Delmonte reported wrongly on PMR in his otherwise very good review). Delmonte showed that there is a rift between improvements on cognitive anxiety and physiological anxiety for meditators. It seems that in fact meditation has more effects on cognitive well being than other interventions.

Holmes (1985, 1987) had argued that studies controlling for placebo variables as 'expectancy' and 'sitting for relief' (Smith, 1976) did not add evidence about superiority of meditation in this respect. Smith (1976) compared three control conditions with TM over a period of four months and found improvements for trait anxiety and physical symptoms equally ameliorated. However, the argument against this study is that the control conditions were *all meditation techniques* in themselves (and not mock-meditations and ruminating on thoughts as referred to by Holmes).

The first was sitting upright and still without meditating, for 20 minutes, identical to Holme's simple resting method. The second and third were in fact forms of concentrative meditation. One focussing even on the powerful Vedic mantra *shanti* whose meaning (peace) most probably had been even known by the subjects in those post flower-power days. The other one was an exercise in positive thinking namely practising "deliberate pursuit [of] a sequence of cognitive activity that has a positive direction and is comprehensive" either fantasy-day-dreaming, storytelling or listing (p.634). One of the three activities had to be chosen and filled with only *positive* contents. It has been noted already that sitting still without doing anything is regarded as a difficult task by meditation experts and that therefore mantras are given as in the second condition. The third condition could also range as a meditation exercise given by an expert of the Hindu or Buddhist tradition. However, he or she would always balance it with a negative exercise because the negative is never denied but dealt with by bringing it to consciousness. For example if imagining the most favoured or loved people was one task the next would have been to imagine those who are most hated. Smith (1987) suggested then to extract meditation skills from the research on meditation in order to employ them for therapy. Very well then, he should acknowledge that those who have invented meditation practices probably had those therapeutic effects in mind when they designed their techniques.[9]

---

[9] C. G. Jung and F. Perls therefore have been inspired by the spiritual traditions of the East

Attrition from meditation or: dropping out

Since stress management research projects always had to deal with subjects dropping out of the treatment period, the question arose whether personality traits were related. Delmonte reported five studies with evidence for drop-outs[10] being more anxious than continuers in cross-sectional studies. Consistent with this was that they scored higher on measures of psychopathology and lower on measures of self-esteem. The results of anxiety reducing effects of meditation could therefore simply be explained by attrition of the more anxious subjects. Since no investigation was conducted with longitudinal design structure *and* strict random allocation to the groups, the question for anxiety reducing effects of meditation could not be satisfactorily answered. However, one study counteracted the problem by using prospective meditators as controls (Van den Berg & Mulder, 1976). Like two other longitudinal studies (see Delmonte, 1987, p.121 for references) these authors found anxiety reduced with meditators but not with controls.

Mood and Stress Management

Peveler & Johnston (1986) tried to investigate the mechanism of those ameliorating long term effects which relaxation and meditation undeniably had on mood states. Their hypothesis suggested that the therapeutic effects of meditation and relaxation could in part be mediated by cognitive and behavioural changes resulting from certain cognitive effects of regular practice. That is because studies on effects of mood on memory could show that mood states are linked to retrieval of memories. Sad thought and memories become more accessible in depressed mood states. The analogy was made that through regular elicitation of a relaxed mood, retrieval of positive cognitive content becomes frequent and changes cognitive and behavioural patterns of the practising individuals. Such cognitive changes can be traced by word lists containing adjectives describing a state of mind or body feeling like e.g. *happy, alert* or *calm* on and place them on a dimension as *distress, arousal* or *appraisal*. Peveler & Johnston (1986) used the adjective checklist of Meddis & MacKay revised by Cruickshank (1984) and found positive changes on the dimensions "arousal" and "distress" in therapy led relaxation sessions and solo practice. Positive effects were also found in the therapist condition with placebo training although solo practice had no effect in the placebo condition.

---

[10] One author used the colloquial short form "drop-outs" and this term will be used to simplify the expression although it sounds a bit disrespectful.

1.8 Hypotheses and Design

1.8.1 Research Design and Paradigm

Two orthogonal research tasks associated to individual differences in the cardiac defense response (Eves & Gruzelier, 1984) followed from the review on research presented in this chapter. One is on correlations between Eysenck's and Strelau's psychometric scales and individual differences in the periods of *long latency* (15-55 s) and *short latency* (1-10 s) post-stimulus. The other was about attenuating effects of progressive muscle relaxation (PMR) as one independent variable on CDR-related reactivity in the periods of anticipation of an auditory stressor of high intensity (Eves & Steptoe, 1989). From that followed an experimental paradigm suitable for the elicitation of both kinds of response pattern (anticipatory and defensive response) similar to the studies reported above with moderate and high intensity stimuli (Figure 1.1). Main dependent physiological variables had to be among others, HR and EMG measures, main dependent psychological variables, among others, the scales of Eysenck and Strelau (EPI, STI). Two physiological experimental sessions were then needed for measuring pre-and post training differences (*between* and *within-subject*) in the dependent variables.

The paradigm of the experiment was as follows: After a resting period of 5 minutes a moderate stimulus of 1 sec duration and 52dB white noise warned the subject of an impending very loud, but not painful noise (110 dB) after a period of 60 seconds. The anticipated high intensity stimulus, however, was actually the presentation of a double stimulus consisting of two 1-sec-stimuli interleaved by a 1-sec inter-stimulus-interval. The subject was not instructed about the exact stimulus design in order to secure a strong reaction due to some novelty effect. The subject was given 2 1/2 minutes of impact and recovery time before the stimulus combination was being repeated with exactly the same temporal characteristics. A schema of the first stimuli presentation is displayed in Figure 1.1. Further information on details and other independent and dependent variables of this experiment are being treated in the task specific paragraph (Clinical Task) further below.

Thus the first experimental session was crucial not only for assessment of the pre-treatment values in the physiological parameters but also for the assessment of individual differences in the two response patterns (anticipatory and defensive). They represented the basis for all further investigation. The personality/temperament task is, logically, therefore directly related to the results of the first session, which does not necessarily mean that the results have to be presented in that order. The hypotheses and further consideration on design structure and variables are found in the following paragraphs. The hypotheses, if not indicated otherwise, refer to heart rate.

Figure 1.1

Paradigm

Moderate Warning Stimulus
52dB, 1 sec duration

High Intensity Double Stimulus, 110dB,
2 x 1 sec, 1 sec inter-stimulus-interval

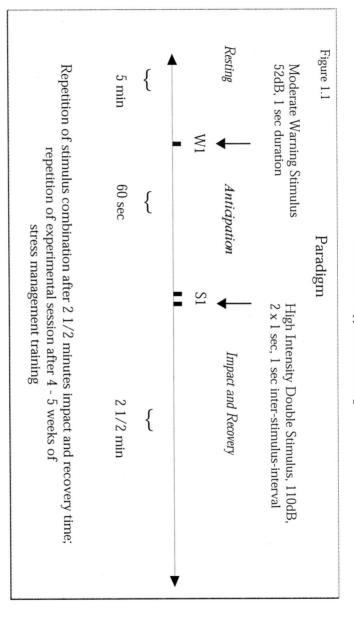

Resting

W1

Anticipation

S1

Impact and Recovery

5 min

60 sec

2 1/2 min

Repetition of stimulus combination after 2 1/2 minutes impact and recovery time;
repetition of experimental session after 4 - 5 weeks of
stress management training

1.8.2 Individual Differences of the Cardiac Defense Response

Individual differences in long latency and reactivity in anticipation, Hypothesis 1

In an experiment employing the above paradigm, individual differences between secondary Accelerators and non-Accelerators in the long latency period post high intensity stimulation (Hypothesis 1.1) could be taken for granted because they had been confirmed several times in different laboratories (e.g. Eves & Sartory, 1989; Richards & Eves, 1990). Anticipatory differences were also expected to occur (Hypothesis 1.2) though not at the same degree of certainty, when it was taken into account that the original findings (Eves, 1984) had been confirmed only in the Eves & Steptoe study. Finally the reflection of long latency differences in the short latency period were to be tested for on this occasion too. Differences over time and in response shape in the acceleratory response peak were expected to occur. EMG-startle referred to the contraction of the neck muscles during the first three seconds post high-intensity-stimulus onset. Differences were predicted that cardiac secondary Accelerators would be exhibiting starker contractions of the neck muscles than non-Accelerators. Other physiological parameters were investigated with regard to CDR-differences as blood pressure, respiration-rate and SCL. Only SCL had been employed in previous investigations (Eves, 1985) but predictions could not be made because the results had been contradictory in different studies.

Dishabituation of CDR after long inter-session interval, Hypothesis 2

In the context of this experimental design another hypothesis with regard to the CDR is being taken to the test for the first time. The question is, whether the rapidly habituating differences of long latency *dishabituate* with an intersession interval of four to five weeks. That hypothesis is important because in case of dishabituation we could expect individual differences in a 'no treatment' control condition. If we consider the secondary acceleration being a part of the "true" defensive response (Eves 1984) then we must assume that dishabituation will be taking place after this long inter-session interval. Therefore, it is expected that individual differences of the long latency period will re-occur after a four to five week's interval in a similar way as in the first session. Dishabituation is considered being a characteristic feature of the defensive response (Sokolov, 1969 and Graham, 1976).

Personality and the CDR, Hypotheses 3

Orthogonal to the clinical task would have been the investigation of correlations between physiological personality measures and the CDR, as had been demonstrated by Richards & Eves (1990). This would have been solely a replication task by analysing the covariations of heart rate with psychometric differences at different levels of analysis. Thus it would have been predicted that Accelerators scored lower on strength of excitation (SE) strength of inhibition (StI), mobility (M) and Extraversion (E) and higher on neuroticism (N). Accordingly low scorers on SE, StI, M and E would have been expected to exhibit a higher heart rate response mean than high scorers. Respectively high scorers on N would have had to exhibit higher heart rate response mean than low scorers (all hypothesis 3). These covariations were also expected to appear in the response shapes of the heart rate changes over time. Finally, since Kline *et al.*, (1993) found smaller auditory evoked potentials (lower amplitude intensity slopes) at intense stimulus levels (94db, 104dB) it was suggested that Lie scores covaried negatively with cardiac responsivity to high intensity auditory stimulation and reversely that secondary non-Accelerators scored higher on Lie scores than secondary Accelerators.

1.8.3 Attenuating effects of Stress Management Methods on CDR related Reactivity, Hypotheses 4

PMR as first experimental treatment condition

Previous research evidence on effects of short term training in progressive muscle relaxation (Eves & Steptoe, 1986) had provided us with evidence for the hypothesis that brief relaxation training reduced anticipatory reactivity related to the cardiac defensive response. The question was whether in an experiment of the same paradigm, high intensity auditory stimulation preceded by a moderate intensity warning (Figure 1.1), with an extended PMR training period of 4-5 weeks, attenuating effects of Accelerator's anticipatory HR and EMG-startle would also occur. It was assumed that the extension of the training period would increase the effects of PMR-training. As had been pointed out the pathways of generalisation process from single muscle groups to the whole motor muscular system were not known, but extension of practising time usually enhanced this process.

Meditation as competing treatment condition

Scarcity of studies with High Intensity Stressors and Initial Measurement

Only a few experiments on effects of stress management have been documented that involved high intensity stressors. The studies by Goleman & Schwartz (1976) and by Lehrer *et al.* (1983) have worked with aversive film sequences in order to test complex emotional stimuli. The latter and Lehrer *et al* (1980) included also auditory tone stimuli of 100 dB intensity and so did the very first study conducted by Orme-Johnson (1973) using a 100dB tone of 3000Hz investigating recovery from stressor impact. However, none of these studies was carried out with repeated physiological measurement (before and after treatment). Lehrer *et al* (1983) argued that responses to laboratory-stressors would strongly habituate with repetition. The downside of that argument is that no initial differences of the physiological variables can be assessed which makes any treatment effects questionable (Holmes, 1984, 1987).

A new meditation technique from the Tantric tradition

The lack of any such adequate study alone justified the implementation of a meditation technique into the design. Given that those few studies have investigated the effects of one single technique only, TM, another technique, perhaps one that had not been under investigation yet, was favourable.

Corby, Roth *et al* (1978) had investigated a technique from the tantric tradition that the authors explained as incorporating the "concepts of energy and energy centre" (*chakra*). They found activating effects and accelerative orienting responses in proficient Tantric meditators and relaxation responses in absolute beginners without training at all. These differences were found during meditative states in response to orienting stimuli and not in response to a stressor. Since there was no study on TM comparing beginners to more proficient meditators of the TM-siddhi technique, it could not be said, whether proficiency or the characteristics of the technique had accounted for these between subject differences. Further: a beginner group with 1-2 months training as in the TM-studies would have had been more useful. Besides, the beginner group had been taken from a college population and not from the institute as the trainees and experts had. Hence self selection could not be excluded as a confounding factor either. Thus for several reasons we were not able to predict, whether tantric meditators would react defensively in anticipation of a high intensity stressor as those TM meditators from the three studies known to us, or, whether they would respond with orienting. Therefore only two-tailed hypotheses could come into question for the variable meditation as a competing method of stress management to PMR.

The other hypothesis put to the test was on recovery from stressor impact. It had to be predicted then that meditators recovered faster from stressor impact than controls and relaxers. However, the first time investigation of this kind of technique required also two-tailed hypothesis.

An active, concentrative meditation technique - Aum Swarupa Dhyan Yoga (ASDY)

TM had often been quoted as a "passive" concentrative technique because of the purely mental activity that is required from the aspirant by repeating a mantra (e.g. Wallace, 1970). A meditation technique that combined several cognitive and physical activities during sitting upright with closed eyes can therefore be regarded as an active technique. The components of the ASDY-technique were:

➢ Physical: Mantra chanting, mainly *Aum*, according to Hindu philosophy the original mantra that all other mantras come from.

➢ Cognitive: Visualizing figures (square, crescent, triangle, wave, circle and dome) related to *chakras* or *energy centres* in particular parts of the nervous system (see Methods section). The meditation process was practised and learnt by:

➢ Physical-cognitive: Listening to a tape-recorded meditation sequence of half an hour, which also gave instructions to the trainee.

The main behavioural difference to TM-practice seemed to Lie in the chanting feature, which served mainly the function of controlled breathing *(pranayama)*. Smith (1978) argued that the de-activating effects of meditation might be linked rather to the sitting position with closed eyes than to the mental mantra activity. In fact, the activities described above were also meant to keep the meditator conscious as explained earlier.

Further: "active" in this context must not be confused with "activating". According to this author's experience the technique has an effect which is difficult to describe. A 15 minutes practice was described by German undergraduates of a pilot study in Hamburg as "simultaneously relaxing and stimulating". The effect of 45 minutes practice is subjectively indeed quite strong and the author of this thesis would perhaps compare it to the condition after coming out of a captivating movie. The effect of an aware but relaxed psychological state may probably come from intense mental activity in different modalities ("multimodal") while sitting in the dark without being physically active. Also: the author of this thesis has witnessed the relaxing effects of this meditation technique over years in group-meditations with young German practitioners.

The ASDY-meditation technique therefore was considered as unsuitable for practice in the experimental chamber before a high-intensity stress experiment. The intensive effects of this meditation technique would not allow being followed directly by a resting period and the remainder of an intense stress experiment. This was regarded as an unethical application of the technique. TM as a less physical and cognitive effort demanding technique clearly had an advantage here.

A meditation session in another room immediately before the experiment would have been a possible alternative from the design point of view. However, a general lack of room facilities in the college where the experiments were conducted, excluded this option to be implemented into the design. Therefore, the design had to rely fully on the effects of daily practice, ideally two times as suggested by the experimenter (see Methods section).

Although this feature made this experiment different from the experiments in the literature, it had an advantage too. Since the technique, because of its intensity, had strong immediate effects on well being of the meditator, it was intriguingly interesting to see what the effects would be after a training period of 4-5 weeks. Moreover, reference to the Eves & Steptoe study is easier since their subjects did their relaxation practice independently and outside the experimental chamber.

Blood Pressure, Respiration Rate, Skin Conductance

In the Goleman & Schwartz study (1976) recovery differences were also found in responsivity of the electrodermal system. Corby, Roth *et al* (1978) found differences in SCL between proficient meditators and absolute beginners, the former being more activated than the latter. Electrodermal activity as an indicator of sympathetic activation in TM-research often demonstrated the activation reducing effects. SCL as a measure of tonic activity therefore had to be included.

By the same token the measurement of diastolic and systolic bloodpressure (DBP, SBP) had to be integrated.

Respiration-rate (RR) was necessary to control for respiratory sinus arrythmia since low breathing rates in combination with high amplitudes result in maximum RSA while the reverse (high rates / low amplitudes) have minimal effects on heart rate (Eckberg, 1983). Apart from that breathing rate has often shown reductions in meditation studies without concomitant heart rate reductions (e.g. Wallace, 1970; Corby, Roth *et al* 1978), which is another reason to employ respiration rate in this study. [11] However, to measure amplitude reliably more sophisticated device would have had to be employed than resources overall would have allowed

Measures of mood state anxiety and ratings of the high intensity stimulus characteristics after the experiment were planned for assessment of subjective states.

---

[11] The cardiovascular effects of pranayama techniques (= controlled breathing) started to come under scrutiny 3 years after the data on this experiment were completed. That research is being discussed in context with the results.

A waiting list control group

Lehrer *et al* (1983) used to argue against repeated measurement with rapid habituation characteristic of stress responses in the laboratory. To avoid confounding effects of this kind, a waiting list control group with no treatment at all implemented into the design.

According to Holmes (1984, 1987) only "simple resting" would have been adequate for measuring activation reducing effects of stress management methods. As explained in the introduction, there is reasonable doubt that such a condition could have been established simply because "simple" resting is not so simple simply because of the uncontrolled cognitive strategies used by the subjects (Shapiro, 1985). Hence, competing relaxation methods of all kinds were regarded sufficiently as control conditions for any technique that claimed to reduce sympathetic activation.

Personality, cognitive variables and stress management group; Hypothesis 5

Right from the beginning of the experiments random allocation to the Stress Management Groups proved a difficult task. That was because many participants resisted 4 weeks daily meditation practice. Although random selection is a requirement for an appropriate experimental design, under given circumstances it was seen as an advantage to assess initial values of self-selected meditators rather than risking a high drop-out rate by talking reluctant participants into meditation practice. The advantage was to look at physiological differences between different stress management choices. One of the critical arguments regarding activation reducing effects of meditation had been that prospective meditators had a lower initial activation level anyway than prospective non-meditators. Therefore it would have been expected that meditators had a lower initial activation level than non-meditators.

Psychological differences on Extraversion, Neuroticism, State Anxiety as described by Delmonte (1987) between self selected meditators, relaxers and controls, could therefore be tested as well as physiological differences and differences of the Nervous System Properties. Thus we would expect prospective meditators being more introvert, neurotic and state anxious than prospective controls. Since Extraversion is correlated with Strength of Excitation (StE) we could expect meditators being lower scorers on StE than controls. Since the hypotheses were derived entirely from research on TM-meditators from which the active features of ASDY-meditation are distinctly different, two tailed hypotheses was applied in the statistic evaluation procedure.

2. Methods

2.1 Subjects

Subjects were 61 male and 40 female mostly students but also some members of technical and teaching staff of Middlesex University, Enfield, in suburban London. They had been recruited by advertisements on student boards all over the campus site and by personal approach. Their average age was 27.1 with a range from 19 to 54 years. None of the subjects suffered from cardiovascular diseases or reported any hearing problems. In addition subjects on cardio-active medication were excluded from the study. They all completed the first experimental session and an introduction into one of the stress management methods if they were not in the no-training control-group.

There were two first session samples. The sample for *tonic* response analysis included all 101 subjects who had participated in the first session before being allocated to the stress management groups. For *phasic* response analysis one more record was incomplete for technical reasons and therefore only 100 records were at hand.

There had been 23 subjects who "dropped out" of the investigation, i.e. they did not appear for the second, post stress-management-training experiment. In addition, three records of the remaining 78 participants were incomplete in a part of the session recordings for technical reasons. So, we had a sub-sample of 75 subjects who completed both sessions and had a complete heart rate record of both sessions. Hence for analysis of both sessions we had 75 records for *tonic*, and 74 for *phasic* responses (see also 2.7).

There were reliably more males than females in both samples: The proportions of male to female in the total sample were (62 : 39; $chi^2(1)=5.24$, p=0.02) and since more females (14) dropped out than males (9) there were more than twice the number of males than females (51 : 24; $chi^2(1) = 10.1$, p<0.01) in the two-sessions- sample. However, the proportions in the two active stress management groups were more balanced (continuers : dropouts = 14: 10 and 17 : 10, $chi^2(1)$ =0.02, p=0.9). The distribution of gender for the categories continuers and dropouts can be seen in Table 2.1.

Table 2.1 Distribution of Gender for Continuers and Dropouts

	Continuers	Dropouts	Total
Male	53	9	62
Female	25	14	39
Total	78	23	101

Because of incomplete data sets one more record was removed from respiration rate, (n=73), four more for analysis of SCL and blood pressure (n=69) and a further two records for analysis of the EMG (n=67).

2.2 Stress Management Training

The training in PMR and in meditation was different in the modes and time points in which the instruction was given. While PMR was trained in a 45 minutes single session with the experimenter, the meditation technique was introduced in a group continuously run on Thursday evenings. Mostly the training in PMR was given directly after the first experimental session but for organisational reasons this could not be maintained for everyone and so the initial training was put on one of the next two days alternatively. The meditation group subjects were instructed to come on Thursday evenings for the group meditation. So, the time gap between the first experiment and the initial meditation training was on average 3 days. The meditation group was asked to do the meditation individually every day or at least every other day and to come for the group meetings once a week. The PMR group was asked to do the training every day and to come for a check-up of the right application of the technique in a group-meeting during the second week. While the meditation group was attended rather regularly, which cannot be said of the PMR-checking group.

2.2.1 Progressive Muscle Relaxation

Like in the Eves & Steptoe study the training in PMR followed a modified version of the "Stanford Behavioural Medicine Relaxation Procedure, Schedule A" (Scheider, Allen *et. al.*, 1980) that included standardised instructions. The participant was seated in a comfortable slightly inclined armchair and the experimenter made sure that the instructions were followed appropriately. The training involved tensing and relaxing the different muscle groups throughout the body and breathing exercises interleaved with the relaxation. At the end of the training session, other than in the reference study but as suggested by the manual, the subject was asked to imagine a Ping-Pong ball on a table tennis surface in a few yards distance. This cognitive relaxation feature was included in order to help the subject to relax the eye muscles. Directly before and after the relaxation training the subject filled in the adjective-checklist

After the session was over a tape of 30 minutes length with the instructions spoken by the experimenter was handed over and the subject was asked to do the exercises once a day and if liked twice.

2.2.2 Aum Swarupa Dhyan Yoga (ASDY) - a complex concentrative Meditation Technique

The concentrative meditation technique followed the guidelines given by the spiritual teacher and ayurvedic physician Dr. Balaji També (També, 1982). It involved a sitting position with eyes closed and chanting of the syllable *Aum*, i.e. to "open up the voice fully and to slide up from the lower note to the basic note" (Vol. 3, p. 47). In another part of the technique other mantras were sung together with the main mantra: *Aum Lam, Aum Vam, Aum Ram, Aum Yam, Aum Ham-Ksham, Aum*. These combined mantras referred to the *chakras*, described by the *Vedas*, the ancient scriptures of the Hindus. The *chakras* are actually assumed energy centres of the body connected to the nervous system and they supposedly also represent psychological centres.

The row of mantras was sung several times and each time in an ascending and descending line according to the rules of the Indian music system *(ragas)*. While singing the meditator was asked to visualize symbols of the chakras: a yellow sqare for *Lam*, a silver crescent for *Vam*, a red triangle for *Ram*, a grey-green wave for *Yam*, a blue circle for *Ham-Ksham* and a bright dome for *Aum*, representing also the mantra of the *sahastradala chakra* at the top of the head.

To make the chanting easier the meditator could use a tape and do the chanting along with the tape. Such meditation tapes were also used during the meditation group meetings. After introduction and meditation was over the first-time-participants were handed over the same meditation tape as just heard. The tape that had been recorded for this experimental purpose, included explanations of the *chakras* and well-known poetry containing paradox images reminiscent of the "sound of one hand clapping". It should be said that the *chakra* theory met, of course, with due academic scepticism on the side of the subjects, but these explanations were given to provide the western minded students with some understanding for the seemingly awkward sounding singing-procedure. In this context also the Vedic understanding of the syllable *Aum* was given as "the first expression of creation" (e.g. També, 1982, 1, p. 4). So the subjects were asked just to do the technique and nothing else. Directly before and after the meditation the subjects filled in the adjective-check-list.

2.3 Stimulus material

The subjects received passive stimulation through headphones with brief moderate and high intensity (loud) white noise. The moderate warning stimulus anteceded the loud one by 60 seconds, and 150 seconds after the loud stimulus compound the sequence was repeated (see paradigm display in section Hypotheses and Design).

The characteristics of the moderate warning stimulus were 57.5 dB white noise with controlled rise and fall time and one second of duration. The loud stimulation was a double stimulus composed of two one-second 110 dB white noise stimuli separated by one second. (All stimuli were coming from a custom built white noise generator calibrated monaurally using a Bruel & Kjaer 2209 sound level meter (A-scale) in conjunction with a Type 4152 artificial ear.) The stimuli were presented over standard audiometric headphones. Stimulus timing and control was achieved with a BBC master micro-computer.

2.4 Apparatus and Physiological Recording

Physiological variables were monitored with a Grass 7D polygraph.

The heart signal was taken from silver plated plate electrodes using EKG lead III. The EKG signal was then transformed into beats per minute averaged heart rate by the cardiotachograph with an AC preamplifier 7P4 and a .03 time constant from the AC amplifier. The transformation implied an error range of +-5%.

Skin resistance was recorded from the medial phalanges of the first and second fingers of the non-preferred hand using Ag/ACl-electrodes of 1cm diameter, and a jelly according to the recommendations made by Fowles, Christie *et al.* (1981). The signal was recorded by a low-level DC preamplifier 7P1 delivering a constant current of 10μA.

For EMG the activity of the semispinalis and splenius muscles in the neck region was recorded with Ag/AgCl cup electrodes attached with double-sided adhesive collars to abraded sites into which electrode jelly had been rubbed, so that resistance between the electrodes was below 10 Kohms. They were placed bilaterally over the mid-points of the unilateral placements recommended in the literature (Lippold, 1967, cit. Schandry, 1989). This placement of electrodes was used by Eves & Steptoe (1989) to avoid contamination of the EMG data with differences in head orientation in which the muscles measured are involved. They referred to pilot work demonstrating "that the integrated activity of the bilateral placements was correlated with the sum of the integrated activity from the two unilateral placements over a 50° and 30° range of head orientations in the horizontal and vertical planes respectively (Spearman's Rho; range = 0.88-0.94)"(p.9). The signal was pre-amplified by a wide band AC preamplifier and integrator 7P3 which cut off the low and high frequencies below 1Hz and above 200Hz. The time constant for integration and amplification was 0.2 and 0.08.

Respiration was measured with a Grass pneumatic respiration transducer (Model PRT) linked to a 7PI DC preamplifier, positioned approximately 5cm below the sternum. Blood pressure was taken from a digital sphygmomanometer monitor working on the basis of the Riva-Rocci principle.

2.5 Questionnaires - Psychological Variables

Personality: For assessment of Extraversion, neuroticism and Lie the Eysenck Personality Inventory (EPI), Form B was applied (Eysenck & Eysenck, 1963). For measurement of properties of the nervous system a questionnaire was copied from the 134 items of the Temperament Inventory presented in Strelau's publication on Temperament, Personality and Activity (1986).

State anxiety: The Self-evaluation questionnaire STAI, Form Y-2 (Spielberger, Gorsuch, Lushene, Vagg & Jacobs, 1977) asks to rate 20 statements on positive and negative feelings "right now, at this moment" on a 4-point scale.

Mood was measured with the Meddis & MacKay adjective checklist revised by Cruickshank (1984) of 18 adjectives pertaining to the factors *arousal, distress* and *appraisal.* The list was given to the subjects before and after training in either of the two types of stress management. (The control subjects had had no training and so there was no control condition for this variable.) The records of 53 subjects were analysed. The adjectives mirroring the mood were measured on a 4-point bipolar scale with the extremes "definitely not" and "definitely", the medium positions were described by "possibly not" and "slightly". Each dimension was measured by the responses to six positive and negative poled adjectives and so the scores for each dimension were between the maximum and minimum scores of $+9$ to -9. The adjectives for *distress* were: tense, worried, uneasy, peaceful, relaxed, calm; for *appraisal* they were: sad, downhearted, gloomy, joyful, pleased, happy; for *arousal*: sleepy, sluggish, drowsy, lively, alert, energetic.

Ratings of noise characteristics: The subjective experience of *loudness* and *unpleasantness* of the high intensity Stimulus only was measured on a seven point rating scale with the anchor points "neutral" and "deafening" for loudness and "neutral" and "very painful" for unpleasantness. Midpoints were "loud" and "unpleasant". This scale was used by Eves (e.g. 1985) for his studies on individual cardiac differences in response to high intensity auditory stimulation.

2.6 Procedure

2.6.1 Course of Experimental Sessions

Each subject participated in two identical experimental sessions, one before and one after training. Due to scheduling problems the inter-session-interval was 4-5 weeks. They had been informed about the aims of the research already in the recruiting phase. After the subjects were screened for heart and hearing problems through a socio-demographic questionnaire the experimenter took blood pressure for the first time. Then they filled in the personality questionnaires (EPI, STI, Spielberger et al.'s state anxiety) which took 25 minutes on average. The electrodes were attached and the subject was led into a sound and light attenuated and temperature controlled laboratory adjacent to the room with the recording apparatus. He or she was seated in a comfortable chair, the respiration belt was attached, and the electrodes were connected to the recording system. Blood pressure was taken for the second time and the recordings of the physiological signals were checked on the polygraph. Then the experimenter entered the chamber again and explained the exact course of the experiment. The subject was informed that after five minutes resting time a discrete moderate intensity noise would be heard over the headphones which would be followed one minute later by another, very loud and unpleasant but not harmful noise. The same sequence would be repeated after a couple of minutes resting time and after a further short time (two minutes recording after stimulation) the experiment would be over. He or she was told to refrain from movement as much as possible and to remain relaxed as much as possible throughout the experiment.

After the experiment was over and the electrodes were removed, blood pressure was taken for the last time. The subject rated on a questionnaire "loudness" and "unpleasantness" of the high intensity noise. Then, according to the allocation to the three conditions, the subject received either training in PMR of 45 minutes or an appointment was made for a session on the same or one of the next two days. The subjects allocated to the meditation group were told to come to the next group meditation meeting that was held regularly on Thursdays at 6 p.m. The subjects of the control group were given an appointment after the second session. After the second session, they were free to choose an introduction to either one of the stress management methods. The course of the second, post training session was the same apart from omitting personality questionnaires.

2.6.2 Inter-session interval

The period between the two experimental sessions varied between 4 to 5 weeks. Two exceptions were made. In one case a meditator subject did not want to continue with the meditation. But he wanted to be helpful for the experimenter and offered a second session after 2 1/2 weeks of training. In two other cases, one in the control and one in the PMR-group, the second session happened after eight weeks because of technical problems on both the experimenter and the subjects' sides. The subject had extended the relaxation training accordingly.

2.7 Physiological Data Reduction

2.7.1 Heart Rate

Data reduction for tonic and phasic analysis

The HR-data were converted from inter-beat-intervals (IBI) into beats per minute (bpm) by the cardiotach with an error range of +-5.07. Heart rate was read from the cardiotach line for tonic response off-line over successive 5-second periods, from 10 s prior to the first warning stimulus until 90 s following repetition of the HI-stimulus. For the phasic cardiac responses a programme averaged all full and partial beats, weighted according to the proportion of the interval occupied by each, within successive seconds post stimulus for 10 seconds (Graham, 1975).

Baselines

Since there were two kinds of stimuli we had two kinds of pre-stimulus baselines. In order to control for respiratory influences on heart rate the pre-Warning baselines were assessed for the period of two full respiratory cycles, but at least for 10 seconds, during the resting period respectively recovery period (post first HI-stimulus impact, see Fig.1.1). A programme for phasic responses did this assessment; *tonic responses* and pre-High Intensity baselines for phasic responses were done by hand. The pre-High Intensity baselines for tonic responses were taken from the last 5-sec-windows of the warning sequences. In this context it is mentioned that one subject's record was excluded from analysis because of extreme influence visible in a parallelism of respiration and cardiotachometer curves throughout his polygraphic chart.

Individual Differences in first period of Long-Latency

The categorization into secondary Accelerators, Decelerators and Equivocals was done after the first experimental session and according to the recommendations given by Eves & Gruzelier (1984). The heart beats of the long latency period after the first High Intensity stimulus (15-50 s post-stimulus onset) were then distributed to four different categories: (a) > 4 bpm above baseline (b) above baseline (c) below baseline (d) < 4 bpm below baseline. Subjects were then by application of a non-parametric one sample test for goodness of fit (Kolmogorov-Smirnow) categorised as secondary Accelerators or Decelerators if the distribution showed both significant deviation towards acceleration or deceleration from a null distribution of 25% of beats in each category and had the greatest percentage of beats in one of the extreme categories. Equivocal subjects were those excluded by these criteria. For analyses, equivocal subjects and Decelerators were combined to one category of *non-Accelerators*. So the procedure resulted into two kinds of cardiac responders, labelled as Cardiac Subgroups (see section 2.8, Statistic) with 45 Accelerators and 55 non-Accelerators regarding the records of all subjects who had participated in the first experimental session.

2.7.2 Other physiological variables: EMG, SCL, Blood Pressure, Respiration Rate

Skin resistance and EMG-data were sampled off-line by the same 5-sec-window procedure as described for heart rate. Skin resistance data were converted into log skin conductance (SC). For EMG data, change scores were computed to control for the between-subject variability in tonic levels of activity as far as the startle-component was concerned. For each of the blood-pressure samples, initial at laboratory entry, resting and post-experimental value (before and after physiological experiment), two measurements were taken with an interval of one minute and averaged. Respiration Rate was taken as the rate of respiration cycles per minute. More explanation of data reduction follows at the start of each result section.

2.8 Statistic

2.8.1 Multivariate Analysis of Variance

For multivariate analysis of the variables (fully factorial MANOVA) two between-subject factors and three within-subject factors were employed: The two between subject factors were Cardiac Subgroup (C.SUBGROUP) for individual differences of the CDR with two levels, (Accelerators / non-Accelerators) and Group of Stress Management (SM-GROUP) with three levels (ASDY-Meditation / Relaxation / no- stress management control). The within-subject factors (Fig. 2) were SESSION with two levels for the two physiological experiments (Session 1 and Session 2), REPETITION with 2 levels for post stimulus sequence (e.g. Warning 1 and Warning 2) and TIME with 12 levels for tonic analysis by 5-sec-windows for 55 s post stimulus including baseline (11 time-points post stimulus offset), and 11 levels for phasic analysis of the ten seconds post stimulus plus baseline (10 time-points post-stimulus), see also 2.7 Physiological Data Reduction). The heart rate time-points of the warning sequences were related to the *resting* and *recovery* baselines. The last values of the warning sequences were baselines for the HI- stimulus periods.

See the analytical design structure for within-subject analysis in Figure 2 overleaf. The analytical factor-terms are written in uppercase. The level structures are elaborated only for one level but are valid also for the right side of the display. The events for the two stimulus intensities were analysed separately therefore they were italicised. The complete scheme is applicable to HR and SCL data. For Respiration Rate and EMG only the Time factor had fewer levels (see sections) on these variables.

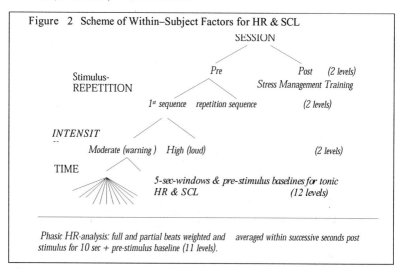

Figure 2 Scheme of Within–Subject Factors for HR & SCL

SESSION

Stimulus-REPETITION

Pre *Post* *(2 levels)*

Stress Management Training

1ˢᵗ sequence   repetition sequence   *(2 levels)*

INTENSIT

Moderate (warning)   High (loud)   *(2 levels)*

TIME

5-sec-windows & pre-stimulus baselines for tonic HR & SCL   *(12 levels)*

Phasic HR-analysis: full and partial beats weighted and   averaged within successive seconds post stimulus for 10 sec + pre-stimulus baseline (11 levels).

For analysis of links between personality measures and tonic and phasic measures of the CDR (baseline, response mean and trends of the polynomial contrasts) multivariate analysis of covariance was employed with a personality measure as covariate and aspects of phasic and tonic heart rate as dependent variables. Further details are given separately at the start of the appropriate result section.

Trend Components of the Polynomial Contrasts as Determinants of Response Shape

The response-shape of a series of heart rate means post stressor stimulus suggests the degree of activation: it is primarily determined by catecholamines ejected into the blood-stream by the adrenal medulla if variance from artefacts like movement and /or breathing can largely be excluded from analysis. Physiologically the differences in response shape matter because frequent cardiac accelerative responding is regarded as a risk factor for cardiovascular disease (Turner, 1994).

Analysis of non-linear trend components (or second order trends) has been used to establish psychological results on levels of physiological activation (e.g. Schandry, 1989), environmental noise (Hays, 1989) or light (Bortz, 1989) optimal for human performance. Howell (1996) in this context also quoted a study on optimal drug dosage for symptom relief. In all cases a positive quadratic curve indicated medium levels of independent variable influence, equidistantly measured on the abscissa (x), for optimal performance measured on the ordinate (y). Such findings are achieved by the method of *orthogonal polynomials* (Winer, 1971) that allots a set of weight coefficients for each trend component tested to the sequence-values of the dependent variable. A trend-component is valid for the heart rate sequence if the sum of variable values exceeds zero (the polynomials alone sum up to zero) and the trend-component of best fit therefore has the largest value (Hays, 1988).

In all studies mentioned above the *successive changes of stimulus strength* dictated the function of the dependent variable sequence as a non-linear trend-component of best fit instead of a simple linear function. Eves & Gruzelier (1984) introduced the method of orthogonal polynomials as a means to analyse *response shapes of heart rate changes over time,* thereby taking the time points of heart rate measurement on the abscissa and heart rate of cardiac subgroups as dependent variable. Such a heart rate sequence following high intensity auditory stimulation necessarily fits a quadratic trend component because of acceleration and deceleration within 10 seconds post stimulus. Equally secondary acceleration necessarily increases the quadratic trend-component, and absence of secondary acceleration will provide a strong cubic trend-component and/or quartic component. Differences in these trend-components will occur if absence and presence of secondary acceleration are the basis for allocation to cardiac subgroups as in the studies with Accelerators, Decelerators and Equivocals of Eves & Gruzelier or with the dichotomic cardiac subgroup category of Richards & Eves and Eves & Steptoe (Equivocals and Decelerators collapsed to non-Accelerators). Therefore differences in all four interpretable trend-components suggest a maximum of difference in response shape. In a nutshell: the higher order trend-components of a series determine the HR-values as functions of the time-axis (x) where directional changes take place and therefore can suggest differences in response-shape of the sequence or (response-curve).

The analysis of shape differences is statistically relevant because the trend components explain more proportion of variance added to the amount of variance explained only by the overall mean differences. The proportion of variance for the differences in mean and all trend-components, i.e. trend components 1-11 for 12 time points, are expressed by Wilks'

Lambda (Λ). We can thus calculate how much of the total variance is explained by reliable differences of mean and interpretable (linear to quartic) trend-components.

Directionality of Hypotheses and Probability of Error

As it has been expressed in the previous section (Hypotheses and Design) directionality of the research-hypotheses were not always one-tailed. This was particularly relevant for the ASDY-meditation technique (referred to also as *active, chanting* or *tantric* technique in the following chapters). All parametric results of the first task of investigation (stress management effects on cardiac subgroups) were evaluated under two-tailed statistical hypotheses. The second task on replicating relationships between CDR and physiologically based personality measures was evaluated under one-tailed hypotheses. The level of significance was chosen with 5% of error probability in both cases. When appropriate, all degrees of freedom from univariate statistics were corrected throughout for spheric violation by the Greenhouse-Geisser coefficient

2.8.2 List of Dependent Variables

Physiological: Heart Rate (HR), Blood Pressure (BP), Respiration Rate (RR), Electromyogram (EMG), Skin Conductance Level (SCL)

Psychological: State Anxiety, Mood, Ratings of High Intensity - Stimulus; Extraversion (E), Neuroticism (N), Lie (L), Strength of Excitation (StE), Strength of Inhibition (StI), Mobility (M).

2.8.3 Partitioning and naming of the measurements over time (time points)

The partitioning of the heart rate variables, (and in fact the variables of Skin Conductance Levels and Electromyogram), followed the stimulus characteristics. Hence the different periods of stimulation, moderate noise for warning and high intensive noise for DR-elicitation, were looked at separately and were labelled as periods of "Moderate Stimulation" or "Warning" (W) and as periods of "High Intensity Stimulation" (S). The measured time points were each indexed by its position in the (post) stimulation sequence. Thus the first heart rate value 5s-post-warning stimulus on-set of the first session was abbreviated as W1(1) and the 11th value of the repetition High Intensity period of the second session was named as $S4_{(11)}$. The values averaged over seconds for the phasic periods were identified by the letters 'ph', e.g '$S1ph_{(1)}$' presents the first second-value post-high-intensity stimulation. The first value BW1ph is the first period baseline value for the phasic Warning time points and BS1ph is the first period phasic High Intensity time point. The time points of measurement are given in brackets in the headings of the analysis section of the heart rate chapter.

3. Results

Introductory Comment

For the main hypothesis, modification of CDR related reactivity by methods of Stress Management, a session comparison was calculated with fully factorial ANOVA (see Fig.2). We had Cardiac Subgroup (C.Subgroup) and Group of Stress Management (SM-Group) as between subject factors and Session, Repetition and Time as within-subject factors (see previous pages for details). Effects involving the single between subject factors have been always reported for analysis with one factor when they appeared significant (p=0.05) in the all-factor-analysis. The same structure was run on the time-points of both types of stimulation, i.e. HI-stimulus and warning, and on the time variables of heart-rate and SCL and for EMG-analysis only different time levels were employed.

Thus, the presentation for the three main variables went first along the stimulus division line. Within stimulus type, sometimes further analyses of the first session was necessary and this is particularly the case for the heart-rate chapter, were events of the first High Intensity sequence were given attention including differences in accelerative peak. That is because the hypotheses on modification of individual differences related reactivity were based on manifestations in the first session. For a similar reason analysis of the first session was extended on the additional records of the drop-out subjects (N=101). Further clarification will be found in the heart rate section.

While the number of heart-rate analyses increased the risk of error, it should be noted, that the additional analyses all relate to hypotheses based on replication of formerly achieved results. Therefore, the danger of type I error is not as serious as it may appear.

3.1 Heart Rate

The session comparison for heart-rate was run on the records of 75 subjects, changes of record numbers in sub-analyses have been indicated appropriately.

What would we expect from the statistics of a comparison of sessions for the events in the HI-stimulus sequences (tonic heart-rate) according to the hypotheses delivered in the previous chapter?

Cardiac Subgroup: We predicted individual differences of secondary acceleration in the long latency period of the first session's first post stimulus sequence habituating within session. We also predicted dishabituation of secondary acceleration in the second session after a 4-5 week's interval for those accelerator-subjects that had not participated in SM-training, i.e. for Accelerators of the Control-Group. Dishabituation would therefore be statistically expressed by an all-factor-interaction of SM-Group X Cardiac Subgroup X Session X Repetition X Time. Such interaction of the between-subject factors would also confound a 4-way interaction effect of Cardiac Subgroup X Session X Repetition X Time even when the Accelerators of Relaxation and Meditation Group were expected to have habituated. Therefore, a clear 4-way interaction as Eves & Steptoe had found (with an inter-session interval of 48 hours) could not be expected. Individual differences of secondary acceleration in long latency as a pre-requisite for the main investigation of SM-effects could therefore only be established by further analysis of the first session's tonic response. This investigation would be incomplete if possible differences in short latency response were not investigated as had been established by Eves & Gruzelier (1984). Analysis of phasic responses therefore has to be included in a separate analysis of these data (see Methods section, data reduction). The analytical procedure for the warning-sequences will be introduced following this section on HI-stimulation.

SM- Group: This factor plays a part on its own apart from its involvement in the main hypothesis, the all-factor interaction already described. One part of that single factor role is not in the original design that intended strictly random allocation to the groups of Stress Management. However, since this issue could not be followed in real life of experimental research, the investigator had to be wary of a selection bias which could be detected by an overall mean effect and/or an SM-Group X Time interaction and indeed in both types of time-variables (HI and Warning). SM-Group could also have session-effects at response-mean level (Session X SM-Group, Session X Repetition X SM-Group) or over Time (Session X Time X SM-Group, Session X Repetition X Time X SM-Group). All these considerations also naturally concern the baselines.

The pre-stimulus baselines (resting and recovery) as reference points had to be tested first. For C.Subgroup no differences were expected, for SM-Group differences were possible in both directions. Hence, interaction effects of SM-Group with one or more of the within-subject factors could be expected.

3.1.1 Sequences post HI- Stimulation, Session Comparison

Baselines, last 5-sec-windows post Warnings, $(W(1-4)_{(12)})$

Between-subjects: There was an effect of C.Subgroup ($F(1,73)=5.41$, $p=0.02$, with one factor; $\bar{X}_{ACCEL}=75.6$bpm, $\bar{X}_{NONACC}=70.8$bpm). There was an effect of SM-Group ($F(2,72)=3.05$, $p=0.05$, $\bar{X}_{Medit}=76.7$bpm, $\bar{X}_{Relax}=71.3$bpm, $\bar{X}_{Control}=71.6$bpm). The differences were reliable between Meditation-Group and both Relaxation and Control-Group ($p<0.05$). There was no interaction of C.Subgroup with SM-Group ($F(2,69)=0.29$, $p<0.75$).

Within-subjects: there was no main effect of Session ($F(1,69)=0.79$, $p=0.38$) but a marginally significant Session X Repetition interaction ($F(1,69)=3.21$, $p=0.08$) suggesting that habituation to repetition of HI-stimulus was greater in the second session ($\Delta W3_{(12)}$-$W4_{(12)}=3.46$) than in the first ($\Delta W1_{(12)}$-$W2_{(12)}=0.36$).

Interactions: There was no interaction of within with between subject factors (Session X C.Subgroup: $F(1,73)=0.31$ $p=0.58$; Session X Repetition X C.Subgroup $F(1,73)=0.41$, $p=0.53$; Session X SM-Group $F(2,69)=0.57$, $p=0.57$, Session X Repetition X SM-Group: $F(2,69)=0.42$, $p=0.45$).

The overall differences in pre-HI-Stimulus baseline of C.Subgroup and SM-Group suggested initial differences since there were no interaction effects with Session. Therefore, one-way ANOVA of the first pre-HI-baseline ($W1_{(12)}$) of the first session was run with the between-subject factors. The hypothesis was not confirmed: There was neither an effect of C.Subgroup ($F(1,69)=1.79$, $p<0.19$) nor of SM-Group ($F(2,69)=0.56$, $p=0.58$). Analysis of both first session pre-HI-baselines (with Repetition added as within-subject factor), however, showed a C.Subgroup main effect ($F(1,73)=4.37$, $p=0.04$) but no C.Subgroup X Repetition effect ($F(1,73)=0.78$, $p=0.38$). There was no effect yet for SM-Group ($F(2,69)=0.63$, $p=0.54$ for SM-Group, $F(2,69)=0.30$, $p=0.48$ for Repetition X SM-Group).

The result for C.Subgroup suggested sensitisation of the Accelerators to repetition of stimulus. The negligible (first) pre-HI-baseline-differences of C.Subgroup ($\Delta W1_{(12)}$ $_{Subgroup}=4.7$bpm) made it possible to look for C.Subgroup differences in the first HI-sequence of the first session. [12] The result for SM-Group suggested that a selection–bias at baseline-level had not taken place.

HI- Sequences, Tonic (W1-4$_{(12)}$, S1-4 $_{(1-11)}$) and Phasic Responses,

Between subject: There was a between subject effect of C.Subgroup ($F(1,73)=8.55$, $p<0.01$; $\overline{X}_{Accel}=74.4$bpm, $\overline{X}_{Nonacc}=69.6$bpm) and no effect of SM-Group ($F(2,69)=1.35$, $p=0.27$) and no interaction of the two factors ($F(2,69)=0.24$, $p=0.8$).

Within subject: There were main effects of Repetition ($F(1,69)=32.3$, $p<0.01$) and Time ($\Delta=0.31$, $F(11,59)=11.74$, $p<0.01$) but no effect of Session ($F(1,69)=0.02$, $p=0.89$). The Repetition effect (built from the averaged means of first and repetition periods from both sessions) indicated habituation to the repetition of the HI-stimulus within a session.

In order to establish the hypotheses on individual differences in *long* and *short* latency, it was first looked at the interactions of the C.Subgroup factor on its own. Results for SM-Group were reported thereafter.

Interactions of Cardiac Subgroup

The hypothesis on habituation of C.Subgroup differences over a session interval of 4-5 weeks was confirmed (Session X Repetition X Time X C.Subgroup: $\Lambda=0.73$, $F(11,59)=1.73$, $p<0.05$). This 4-way interaction suggested individual differences in one of the four HI-sequences and there was no involvement of Stress Management in these differences ($\Lambda=0.71$, $F(22,118)=1.02$, $p=0.45$ for C.Subgroup X SM-Group X Session X Repetition X Time effect).

First Session (W1-2(12), S1-2(1-11))

In order to confirm individual differences of the CDR in first session's first HI-sequence the time variables of the first session were analysed with Repetition and Time as within subject factors and C.Subgroup as between subject factor. An all-factor interaction was expected for the hypothesis. There were main effects of all factors (C. Subgroup: $F(1,73)=7.57$, $p<0.01$; Repetition: $F(1,73)=13.09$, $p=0.001$; Time: $\Lambda=0.31$, $F(11,63)=12.77$, $p<0.001$). There was indeed a 2-way interaction of C.Subgroup X Time ($\Lambda=0.65$, $F(11,63)=3.10$, $p<0.01$) and the desired 3-way interaction effect of C.Subgroup X

---

12 Otherwise the resting baselines could have served as reference points. Those will be investigated later in context with the warning sequences.

Repetition X Time (Λ=0.75, F(11,63)=1.93, p=0.05) suggesting differences in the first HI-sequence.

First Session, First HI-Sequence (W1(12), S1(1-11))

There was a main effect of C.Subgroup (F(1,73)=8.50, p<0.01) and a Time main effect: (Λ=0.29, F(11,63)=14.08, p<0.001) and there was a C.Subgroup X Time interaction (Λ=0.67, F(11,63)=2.80, p<0.01) reflected in the quadratic (F(1,73)=11.96, p=0.001) and cubic (F(1,73)=9.23, p<0.01) trend.

Differences in quadratic and cubic trend together indicated different directions of response over time within the two C.Subgroup sequences. While the quadratic trend reflected predominantly acceleration in one Subgroup's sequence, i.e. in Accelerators, the cubic trend accounted for the decelerative trend of the other cardiac Subgroup's sequence; see Fig. 31.1 overleaf.

Figure 31.1

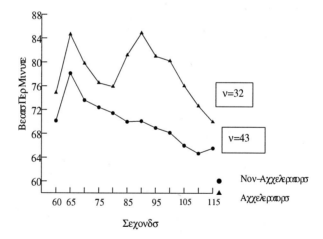

The C.Subgroup X Time differences of the multivariate statistics explained 67.2% of the total variance (see Λ). The C.Subgroup differences of the mean only explained 10.4% of the model variance and the two models for differences in quadratic and cubic trend (response shape) together explained 27.6%.

First HI-Sequence, W1(12), S1(1-11), N=101

Our separate task on CDR related differences in personality measures demanded analysis of the complete first-session-sample. Furthermore, the sample of the subjects who had completed both experiments was selected by attrition and finally: no sample of this size had been investigated before for individual differences in long latency.

So, ANOVA was run with C.Subgroup as between subject factor and Time as within subject factor on the time-variables of the first HI-stimulus sequence of the full first session's sample. There was a main effect of C.Subgroup $(F(1,99)=18.0, p< 0.001, \overline{X}_{ACCEL} = 79.6, \overline{X}_{NONACC} = 70.3)$ and a main effect of Time $(\Lambda= 0.31, F(11,89)=17.79, p<0.001)$. Furthermore the between-subject factor interacted with Time $(\Lambda=0.67, F(11,89)=3.97, p<0.001)$ and this interaction was reflected in differences of the quadratic $(F(1,99) = 22.11, p<0.001)$ and cubic trend $(F=9.22, p=0.003)$. First, see the differences in response-shape in the same format as before for the two-session-complete sample, Fig. 31.2a.

Figure 31.2a

Heart Rate: Tonic Response to High Intensity Stimulation at 60s, First Session
- Accelerators vs Non-Accelerators, N=101

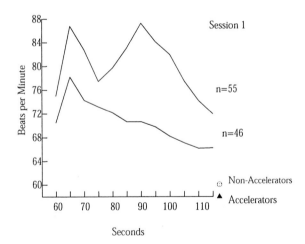

The different directional changes of the Subgroups' heart-rate sequences are illustrated by the trend differences in Figure 31.2b on the next page. For this figure heart-rate was calculated for change scores from baseline. The time scale was based on the 5-sec-windows as in 31.2a. Each Subgroup's heart-rate sequence (triangle for Accelerators, circles for non-Accelerators) is depicted with its quadratic and cubic trends that were both reliably discriminating between C.Subgroups.

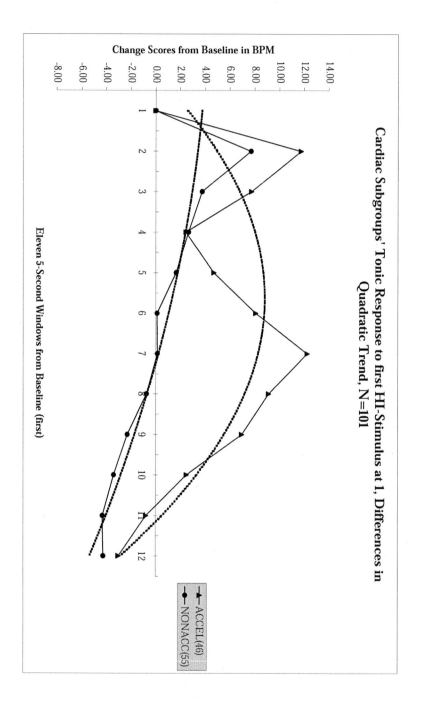

Cardiac Subgroups' Tonic Response to first HI-Stimulus at 1, Differences in Quadratic Trend, N=101

Eleven 5-Second Windows from Baseline (first)

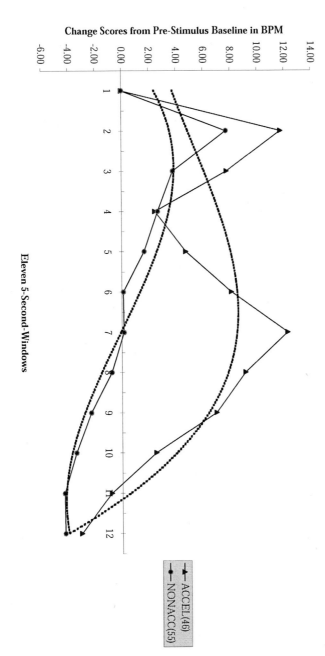

Cardiac Subgroups' Tonic Response to HI-Stimulus at 1, Difference in Cubic Trend, N=101

Change Scores from Pre-Stimulus Baseline in BPM

Eleven 5-Second-Windows

ACCEL(46)
NONACC(55)

First HI-Sequence, N=101, Phasic Response, B1Sph, S1ph (1-10)

Analysis of the tonic responses had shown occurrence of differential heart-rate changes in the period of long latency. Now we had to look at the short latency period for phasic changes within 10 seconds post-stimulation and for this analysis another set of data was used which was based on second-by-second weighted sampling (see Methods, Data Reduction). Previous research, let the differences of the long latency period expect to be mirrored in the short latency response (Eves & Gruzelier, 1984). This would have been indicated by interactions of the C.Subgroup factor with Time.

There was a between-subject effect of C.Subgroup (F(1,99)=12.24, p=0.001, $\bar{X}_{ACCEL}$=86.08bpm, $\bar{X}_{NONACC}$=76.16bpm), a main effect of Time (Λ=0.21, F(10,90) =33.18, p<0.001) and an interaction of C.Subgroup X Time (Λ=0.80, F(10,90)=2.31, p=0.02). These Time differences in the Subgroup factor were reflected in the polynomial contrasts with a quadratic (F(1,99)=10.02, p<0.01) and a cubic trend (F(1,99)= 8.06, p<0.01) indicating that the two C.Subgroups' heart-rate changes differed not only by magnitude over time but also in their response shape. The more responsive cardiac Subgroup accelerated by 21bpm on average from 74.3bpm to 95.7bpm while their counterparts augmented the frequency of their beats per minute only by 11 on average, from 70.22bpm to 81.52bpm. The directional differences are shown in Fig. 31.3

Figure 31.3a

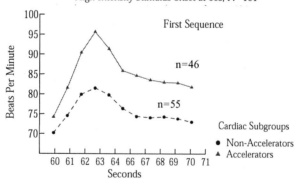

Heart Rate: Cardiac Subgroups' Phasic Response to High Intensity Stimulus onset at 60s, N=101

Accelerative Peak

The difference of response shape in the short latency period reflecting the differences of the long latency period can be given further additional weight by analysing the peaks of acceleration (Eves & Gruzelier, 1984). That is because differences of the first two seconds would be attributable to startle (Graham, 1979). Moreover, by relating each heart beat to its pre-stimulus baseline before the analysis with grouping factors, minor baseline differences from the Resting baseline can be "teased out".

Therefore the individual response profiles of the first ten seconds were at first examined in order to identify the period in which most of the subjects had their accelerative peak. According to previous research and the Ph.D. studies of Eves (1985) this is usually the period between the 2nd and the 4th second. In fact, fairly consistent with Eves' studies (86%), 83 out of 101 subjects (83.8%) exhibited their peak acceleration within this period. Interestingly, however, out of the remaining 18 subjects, 17 displayed their accelerative peak in the period between 6-10 seconds and only one subject in the first second post stimulation. This is surprising if we consider the white noise and fast rise-time characteristics of the double-stimulus: both would be expected to enhance startle acceleration within the first 2 seconds compared to tones (Graham 1979, Hatton et al. 1970). However, we are less surprised if we consider, that with double stimulation within three seconds, the startle reflex measured in the first seconds post offset is very likely to be confounded by habituation.

Figure 31.3b

Phasic Heart Rate, Peak Differences between Cardiac Subgroups

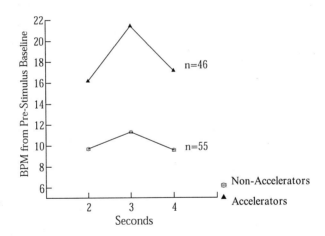

So, the change scores from the respiratory linked baseline of the heart-beats falling into the period between 2nd to 4th second post stimulus on-set were calculated. Then the three change scores were analysed with Subgroup as between-subject and Time as within-subject factor: There were main effects of Subgroup (F(1,99)=19.44, p<0.001, $\overline{X}_{ACCEL}$=18.2, $\overline{X}_{NONACC}$=10.2,) and Time (Λ=0.63 F(2,98)=28.75, p<0.001) and an interaction (Λ=0.88 F(2,98)=6.61, p=0.002) mirrored in the quadratic trend (F(1,99)=13.35, p<0.001), indicating that the heart-rate means of the C.Subgroups took different directions in their peak phases as it is shown in Figure 31.3b above.

Interactions of SM-Group

HI- Sequences, Tonic Response continued (W1- $4_{(12)}$, S1- 4 $_{(1-11)}$)

At the beginning of this section it was reported that there had been no differences of SM-Group in the overall mean. The interaction nearest to an effect was that for Session X SM-Group ($F(2,72)=2.01$, $p=0.14$). Since we had overall mean differences of SM- Group in pre-HI-stimulus baseline, post-hoc tests of hypothesis was run in order to reveal the tendency of session changes. Reliable Session X SM-Group differences between Meditation and Relaxation Group were found ($F(1,49)=4.04$, $p=0.05$). The Meditators had an increase of their second session mean ($\Delta \bar{X} =3.24$bpm), the Relaxers, in contrast, a reduction ($\Delta \bar{X}=-2.47$bpm). The Controls had reduced too by a lesser margin ($\Delta \bar{X}=-0.5$bpm).

HI-Sequences, Phasic Response (Bph1-4, Sph1-4$_{(1-10)}$)

There was a between subject effect of SM-Group in the overall mean ($F(2,71)=3.75$, $p=0.03$) with mean differences between Meditation on top and Control Group at the bottom ($\bar{X}_{MEDIT}=82.9$, $\bar{X}_{CONTROL}=74.7$, Tukey $p<0.03$; $\bar{X}_{RELAX}=76.6$). The interaction for Session X Time X SM-Group confirmed the results from tonic analysis ($\Lambda=0.64$, $F(20,118)=1.45$, $p=0.11$). See Fig. 31.4 a,b, overleaf.

Figure 31.4a

Heart Rate, Stress Management Groups' Phasic Responses
to HI-Stimulus onset at 0 s, Averaged means; N=74.

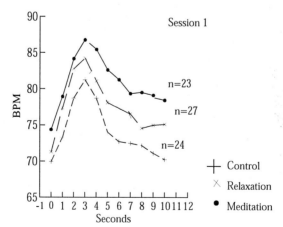

Pre-stimulus baseline from two full respiratory cycles but at least from 10 s resp. activity

Figure 31.4b

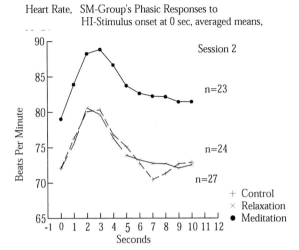

Heart Rate, SM-Group's Phasic Responses to
HI-Stimulus onset at 0 sec, averaged means,

There was no Session main effect ($F(1,71)=0.02$, $p=0.9$) and no Session X SM-Group interaction at mean ($F(2,71)=1.52$, $p=0.23$) or Time level ($\Lambda=0.68$, $F(20,124)=1.30$, $p=0.19$ for SM-Group X Session X Time). There was a near interaction effect with Repetition ($F(2,71)=2.29$, $p=0.11$, for SM-Group X Repetition; $F(1,68)=18.24$, $p<0.001$, for main effect), which had not been observed in the first session's analysis and thus it was looked into the time variables of the second session.

Figure 31.4c   Heart Rate: SM-Groups' Phasic Responses
to High Intensity Stimulation, Means for all 4 Sequences, N=75

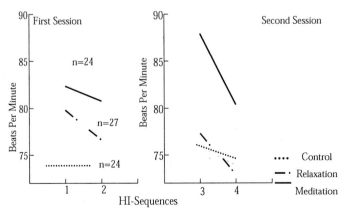

SM-Group X Repetition effect in second Session

Second Session: ANOVA showed an overall mean effect of SM-Group ($F(2,71)$=5.55, p< 0.01) and a Repetition effect ($F(1,71)$=28.47, p<0.01) interacting with each other at the borderline of significance ($F(2,71)$=3.01, p=0.056). Tukey's Multiple Comparison proved significant mean differences between the Meditation Group with the largest ($\overline{X}$=83.7) and the two smaller means of the other SM-Groups (Relaxation: $\overline{X}$=74.7, p<0.01, Control: $\overline{X}$=74.6, p<0.02). See Fig 31.4c, means for second session.

However, the SM-Group X Repetition differences were of a different kind: The Meditators had slightly larger mean differences between the two sequences than the subjects of the other SM-Groups ($\Delta \overline{X}_{MED}$=3.69, $\Delta \overline{X}_{REL}$=2.26, $\Delta \overline{X}$=1.02) and the difference with the Control Group was significant (p=0.04, Tukey's Test). The Meditators had reduced their mean in the Repetition sequence more than the Control subjects.

3.1.2 Sequences post Warning of impending HI- stimulus

Again, it was mainly looked for interactions of the between-subject factors with Session. We had two hypotheses about the events in these sequences of anticipating the impending HI-stimulus. One was about C.Subgroup differences present throughout the time variables of the first session (assumption of sensitising processes) and that would have been expressed by a Session X Time X C.Subgroup interaction effect. For the events in the second session C.Subgroup differences would have been expected only in the time variables of the Control Group because of their attenuation by Stress Management training in the other two groups. That would have found its statistic expression in either an all-factor interaction in the multivariate statistics (if differences were found in one of the sequences similar to Eves & Steptoe) or in a 4-way Session X Time X C.Subgroup X SM-Group interaction effect. The hypothesised effects of the first session were of course the basis for the hypothesised effects in the second session. These effects could have also found expression in the univariate statistics at response mean level (all interactions without Time-factor) but not necessarily. Differences over time are not always reflected by differences in the overall mean, which is why the Time factor was employed. C.Subgroup differences were expected, but SM-Group differences were not unlikely to happen if the expected attenuating impact on anticipatory reactivity had been robust enough.

Before we could run the all-factor analysis on the time variables of Warning, the resting baselines (before first Warning (W1)) and recovery baselines (before repetition (W2)) had to be checked for changes over Session (any interaction of between-subject factors with Session). ANOVA on baselines was run, of course, without the Time factor.

Baselines, Resting and Recovery, (B1-4)

There were no between-subject effects for C.Subgroup ($F(1,69)$=1.30, p=0.26) or SM-Group ($F(2,69)$=0.77) or for interaction of both ($F(2,69)$=0.21, p=0.81). There was no Session effect ($F(1,69)$=1.97, p=0. 16) but there was a Repetition effect because of habituating repetition values ($F(1,69)$=7.42, p<0.01, $\Delta_{B1B3-B2B4}$=2.9bpm).

There was no interaction of C.Subgroup with the within-subject factors ($F(1,69)=0.01$, $p=0.93$ for Session X C.Subgroup) but there was a 3-way interaction effect of SM-Group ($F(2,69)=4.37$, $p<0.02$ for Session X Repetition X SM-Group).

Post- hoc test revealed that the effect occurred due to differences in recovery from HI-stimulus impact between Meditation and Control Group, ($F(1,46)=11.54$, $p=0.001$, $\Delta \bar{X}_{MEDIT} = 3.84$, $\Delta \bar{X}_{CONTROL} = .1.22$), and furthermore, to differences between the Relaxation ($\Delta \bar{X}_{RELAX}=1.64$) and the Control Group ($F(1,49)=4.33$, $p=0.04$). That means, the baselines of both Groups of Stress Management had recovered reliably different from the first HI- stimulus in the second session than the baselines of the no-Stress Management Control Group. Table 31.4 shows the baseline changes in both sessions for SM-Group. Obviously the Meditators had a session shift in resting baseline ($\Delta B_1 B_3=-5.7$bpm) in contrast to the other groups, which suggested some regression to the mean in recovery baseline of Session 2.

Table 31.4: Resting and Recovery Baselines (Means & SE) within Groups; Session X Repetition effect for all and Session effect for Resting (*)

	Session 1				Session 2			
SM-GROUP	B1*		B2		B3*		B4	
Meditation	68.1	2.33	67.7	2.33	73.8	1.78	69.9	1.98
Relaxation	69.3	2.19	67.7	2.20	69.0	1.68	67.4	1.87
Control	68.4	2.33	66.0	2.33	68.4	1.78	69.3	1.98

Warning Sequences, Tonic Response, B1-4, W1-4 (1-11)

ANOVA with both between–subject factors (SM-Group, C.Subgroup) and the within subject factors (Session, Repetition, Time) showed at overall mean level no effect for SM-Group ($F(2,69)=0.88$, $p=0.42$). There was a reliable effect for C.Subgroup ($F(1,73)=5.00$, $p=0.03$, for one factor analysis) but no interaction effect of the two ($F(2,69)=0.12$, $p=0.89$).

There was no effect of Session ($F(1,69)=2.26$, $p=0.14$; Time effect: $\Lambda=0.30$, $F(11,59)=12.26$, $p<0.001$) and there was no effect for the first hypothesis C.Subgroup differences overall in first session ($\Lambda=0.79$, $F(11,59)=1.46$, $p=0.17$ for Session X Time X C.Subgroup; $\Lambda=0.86$, $F(11,59)=0.86$, $p=0.59$ for Session X Repetition X Time X C.Subgroup.

Unsurprisingly then, there was no effect to confirm the second hypothesis either - impact of SM on C.Subgroup differences in second session (Λ=0.76, F(22,118)=0.81, p=0.71 for Session X Time X SM-Group X C.Subgroup; Λ=0.72, F(22,118)=0.94, p=0.54 for Session X Repetition X Time X SM-Group X C.Subgroup).

These findings could have suggested that SM had had no impact on heart-rate and therefore it was looked for overall differences of C.Subgroup. However, there was no effect for C.Subgroup X Time (Λ=0.80, F(11,59)=1.34, p=0.23). So, there was no anticipatory reactivity related to secondary acceleration in any of the four warning sequences, which Stress Management could have had an impact on.

Further analysis however, revealed an interesting interaction at mean level. There was a main effect of Repetition (F(1,69)=8.69, p<0.01, Δ=-3.9bpm) and a Session X Repetition interaction effect (F(1,69)=9.92, p=0.02) because in session 2 the repetition mean (second warning sequence) habituated more than in session 1 (ΔSESSION1=-0.3bpm, ΔSESSION2=-3.6bpm). There was a powerful Repetition effect in the second session (F(1,73)=24.52, p<0.001) as a consequence of the response mean shift ($\overline{X}W_1$=71.5bpm, $\overline{X}W_3$=75.1bpm, p<0.02) in the second session's initial warning sequence ($\overline{X}$ B3 (W3(1-11)).

The baseline session shift of the Meditation Group let expect a 3-way interaction with SM-Group at this level but that was not the case (F(2,69)=1.07, p=0.35 for Session X Repetition X SM-Group). A look at the standard errors of the means suggested changes in variability over session between the groups and that will follow after the presentation of the phasic responses (*see Epilog*).

Instead of SM-Group differences there was a marginally significant interaction effect of Session X Repetition X C.Subgroup (F(1,73)=3.37, p=0.07; see Fig. 31.6). The difference was found in the C.Subgroups' response mean of the first session: the Accelerators *sensitised* to repetition of warning by 1.6 bpm, the non-Accelerators, in contrast *habituated* by almost the same margin (1.7bpm, Session 1: Δ_{W1W2}=0.29bpm). In the second session both cardiac Subgroups habituated with repetition (Session 2: Δ_{W3W4}=3.6bpm; see Fig. 31.5).

Figure 31.5

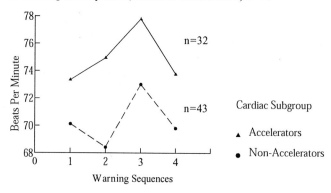

Heart Rate: Cardiac Subgroups' Tonic Response
to Warning and Repetition, Means of both Sessions, N=75

n=32

n=43

Cardiac Subgroup

▲ Accelerators

● Non-Accelerators

Before we continue investigating session interaction effects of the between subject factors in the tonic warning time-variables, a thorough look at the first session events has to be done for the following reasons:

The overall SM-Group differences suggested SM-Group differences in the first session. Stress Management training during the session interval confounded the results of the session-comparison for C.Subgroup differences. The Session X Repetition X C.Subgroup effect suggested C.Subgroup differences in the response mean of the repetition sequence and there had been C.Subgroup X Time differences found at 20% error probability. Both effects raised curiosity about the events in the first session. Furthermore: Finding C.Subgroup differences in the sequences of Warning was not only a pre-requisite of this study but also a replication task of Eves & Gruzelier (1984) as the CDR of long and short latency post HI-auditory stimulation was. Therefore an analysis of the first session's sample unselected by dropping out (N=100) was conducted with the within subject factors Repetition and Time and the between subject factors SM-Group and C.Subgroup. Since we had no interaction effect in the grand analysis the two factors were investigated separately.

Interactions of C.Subgroup in First Session, N=100 (B1, W1(1-11), B2, W2(1-11))

First it was looked at mean level. There was an effect of C.Subgroup (F(1,98)= 5.02, p=0.03, $\bar{X}_{ACCEL}$=75.4bpm, $\bar{X}_{NONACC}$=70.2bpm) and an interaction of C.Subgroup X Repetition (F(1.98)=3.95, p=0.05, $\Delta \bar{X}_{ACCEL}$=1.30 $\Delta \bar{X}_{NONACC}$=-1.89) suggesting sensitisation for the Accelerators and habituation for the non-Accelerators. Consequently there was no main effect of Repetition (F(1,98)=0.038, p=0.85).

Figure 31.6

HR, Cardiac Subgroups' Tonic Response to Warning with Repetition at 0 sec, Averaged Means, Differences, Mean: p=.03, Trends: Linear p=.06, Quadratic p=.07 , N=100

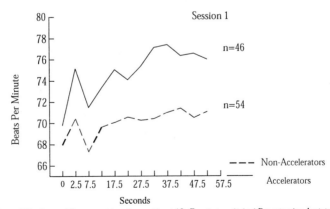

Baselines of Resting and Recovery taken from at least 10s Respiratory linked Pre-stimulus Activity

At time level (Time effect: Λ=0.50, F(11,88)=7.87, p=0.001) we found a C.Subgroup X Time interaction effect in the univariate analysis (F(6,659)=2.27, p=0.03) but only a marginally significant effect in the multivariate statistics (Λ=0.83, F(11,88)=1.65, p=0.095)

mirrored by marginally significant differences in linear $(F(1,98)=3.56, p=0.06)$ and quadratic trend $(F(1,98)=3.37, p=0.07)$ that suggested the slightly more accelerative response shape of the Accelerators superimposed over the C.Subgroup response mean differences, see Fig. 31.6 above.

There was no effect for the interaction of C.Subgroup X Repetition X Time $(\Lambda=0.97, F(11,88)=0.27, p=0.99)$; nevertheless, the two sequences are depicted in Fig. 31.7a,b in order to show the sensitising trend with repetition that accounted for most of the mean differences.

Figure 31.7a Cardiac Subgroups' Tonic Response to first Warning at 0 sec, N=101

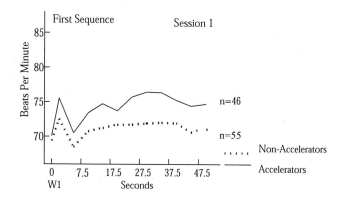

Figure 31.7b   Heart Rate: Cardiac Subgroups Tonic Response to Repetition of Warning at 205 sec

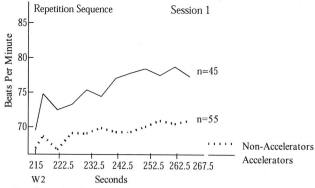

Recovery Baselines taken from at least 10 s respiratory linked activity pre-stimulus

So, we had found some evidence for response shape differences of the C.Subgroups overall in the first session. Additionally the Repetition X C.Subgroup interaction suggested C.Subgroup differences of the mean in the repetition sequence (Fig. 31.7a,b). Analysis of the repetition sequence confirmed a main effect of C.Subgroup (F(1,98)=8.09, p<0.01) and a near interaction effect with Time in the multivariate statistics (Λ=0.81, F(11,88)=1.61, p=0.11) mirrored in a borderline interaction effect with the linear trend in the polynomial contrasts (F(1,98)=3.71, p=0.057). The events of the repetition period (Fig. 31.7b) contributed most to the interaction of the C.Subgroup factor with Time in the heart-rate variables of the first session's warning sequences overall, i.e. averaged means.

Interactions of SM-Group in First Session

It was then looked at whether the SM-Group X Time effect from the two session complete sample persisted in the century sample of the first session (N=100). Interestingly, that was not the case. There was nothing like an effect for SM-Group X Time (Λ= 0.77, F(22, 174)=1.12, p=0.33). The "drop-outs" were from a different population than the continuing subjects were and that will be investigated further in the appropriate section on attrition from Stress Management.

Session analysis continued (Warning, tonic response)

Nevertheless, it was possible that SM did have an effect on heart rate irrespective of the C.Subgroup factor. There was a Time X SM-Group effect overall (Λ=0.59, F(22,124)=1.71, p<0.04) but post-hoc test of hypotheses did not show significant results for any of the three Group comparisons. The time-differences between Relaxation and Meditation Group came nearest to the size of an effect (Λ=0.68, F(11,39)=1.69, p=0.11, Fig. 31.8a,b). In the same post-hoc analysis a Session X Time X SM-Group effect at the borderline of significance was found (Λ=0.64, F(11,39)=2.01, p=0.055) and analysis of the first session showed a marginal SM-Group X Time effect (Λ=0.63, F(22,124)=1.50, p<0.09). Post-hoc test confirmed differences between Meditation and Control Group reliable at the borderline of significance (Λ=0.62, F(11,36)=1.97, p=0.057). This time effect was reflected by the linear (F(1,46)=4.38, p=0.04) and cubic trend-component (F(1,46)=3.91, p=0.05) suggesting response-shape differences. The prospective Meditators developed the most accelerative response and the Controls the most decelerative in both latencies post warning (see Fig 31.5a). The reliable SM-Group X Time effect across sessions was thus a result of these a priori differences of the first session between Meditation and Control Group and of differences between Relaxation and Meditation Group in the second session (Fig.31.8a,b). The latter were largely a consequence of the Meditators' session shift of resting baseline.

Figure 31.8a

Heart Rate: SM-Groups' Tonic Response to Warnings (averaged means), N=75
at 0 sec - Differences over time between Meditation and Control Group (P=0.057)

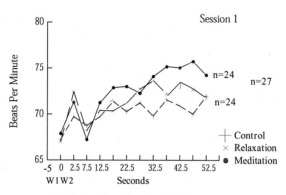

Resting baseline taken from 2 full respiratory cycles

Figure 31.8b   Heart Rate: SM-Groups' Tonic Response to Warnings at 0 sec,
averaged means, N=75

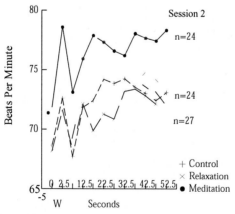

Session X Time X SM-Group effect between meditators and relaxers p<0.055

Warning Sequences, Phasic Response, N=74

The session analysis concludes with the phasic responses to warning as dependent variables. The baseline shift was likely to have had an impact here too.

There was a 3-way interaction of SM-Group X Session X Repetition at response-mean level (F(2,71)=4.74, p=0.01). (Main effects: for Session F(1,71)=4.57, p=0. 04; for Repetition (F(1,71)=8.11, p<0.01; for SM-Group (F(2,71)=1.16, p=0.32).

Post-hoc test confirmed differences between Meditation and Control Group (F(1,45)=9.14, p<0.01) and between Meditation and Relaxation Group (F(1,48)=5.74, p=0.02). The Meditators habituated starkly in the repetition sequence (Δ $\overline{X}_{MED}$=-5.66) following the baseline session shift. The Controls and Relaxers in contrast had both lighter repetition changes but in different directions: the Controls had sensitised slightly (Δ $\overline{X}$=0.62) and the Relaxers habituated (Δ $\overline{X}_{REL}$=-1.06, see Figure 31.9).
Figure 31.9

Heart Rate: Stress Management Groups' Phasic Response Means
to Warning Stimulus with Repetition, both Sessions, N=73

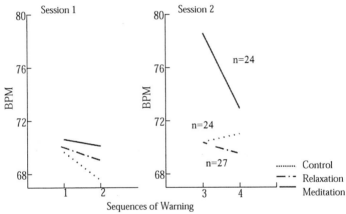

Sequences of Warning
SM-Group X Session X Repetition effect between Meditation
and both Control (p=0.01) and Relaxation Group (p<0.02)

There had been no 5-way effect at Time level for this effect. Nevertheless there was an interaction effect in the averaged means for Session X Time X SM-Group (Λ=0.63, F(20,124)=1.64, p=0.05). The Time differences between Groups over Session is shown in Fig. 31.10a,b. The two stimulus sequences of each session are collapsed by showing the averaged response over ten seconds.

Figure 31.10a

Heart Rate: SM-Groups' Phasic Response at 0 sec
to Warning and Repetition, Averaged Means,

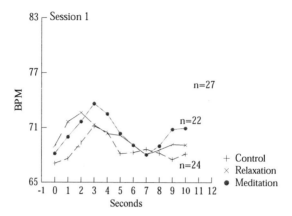

Figure 31.10b

Heart-Rate: SM-Groups' Phasic Response to Warning Stimulus with
Repetition, onset at zero seconds, averaged means, N=73

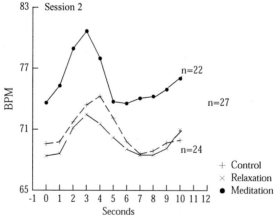

Session X Time X SM-Group differences between Meditators and Controls,
baseline taken from two full respiration cycles, but at least over 10 seconds.

Matched sample comparison

In the first session, the Control subjects had been much better at habituating to the warning stimulus than the prospective stress-management trainees, as can be seen in the linear differences of the first session in Fig. 31.9. The effect suggested that Relaxation and Meditation did have an attenuating effect in the repetition sequence. However, the Meditators had reliably elevated resting-baselines in comparison to both other Groups and therefore the habituation effect was very likely to be a consequence of regression to the mean or law of initial value respectively. In order to test this hypothesis, 10 subjects of each Group were matched on the second session's resting baseline (B3) =< 71.5 bpm and then analysed with the same factors as the whole sample. If the Session X Repetition effect for SM-Group "survived" this operation then regression to the mean could be excluded and Meditation training was more likely to be the cause for the effect. However, the result was negative: There were main effects of Session ($F(1,27)=7.28$, $p=0.01$) and Repetition ($F(1,27)=4.05$, $p=0.05$) and no interaction with the SM-Group factor ($F(1,27)=0.81$, $p=0.45$, $F(2,27)=0.96$, $p=0.40$ for SM-Group main effect).

The overall Session X Time differences between Meditation and Control Group were marginally reliable only ($\Lambda=0.66$, $F(10,36)=1.84$, $p<.09$; Meditation vs. Relaxation Group: $p<0.16$).

Conclusion

Summarising the results of the analysis it has to be said: The hypothesis on individual differences in anticipatory reactivity related to the cardiac defense response was not confirmed. Consequently, we could not find any impact of Stress Management on cardially higher responsive subjects. Moreover, there was no clear evidence for reactivity attenuating effects of any of the methods either. For the active multimodal concentrative Meditation technique, by tendency, anticipatory responsivity was even heightened, expressed by a baseline session-shift and differences over Session and Time in the averaged means of warning.

Epilog: Variability Changes post SM-training blocking effects ? Warnings revisited: Tonic Response

In the analysis of the warning sequences we wondered about a "missing" Session X Repetition X SM-Group effect since the Meditators had a baseline shift in the first sequence of the second session and we had a stark repetition effect there (see second paragraph prior to Fig. 31.5). Therefore a SM-Group difference on the mean or over time should have occurred in that sequence. Thus in order to get a clearer picture of the events ANOVAs of the second session's sequences were run and then it was looked at a session change of variability between Groups in order to find a systematic "effect" that could have "blocked" session effects in the means.

Second Session (B3, W3(1-11) B4, W4(1-11))

First Sequence: Analysis with SM-Group and Time as factors revealed marginal between-subject differences ($F(2,72)=2.86$, $p=0.06$). Tukey's test ($p=0.08$) confirmed differences between Meditators and Relaxers ($\overline{X}_{Medit}=79.2$bpm, $\overline{X}_{Relax}=72.9$bpm).

Repetition Sequence: Analysis had a Time X SM-Group interaction effect (Λ=0.59, F(22,124)=1.72, p=0.03) reflected by the quartic trend-component (F(2,72)=3.12, p=0.05). Post-hoc comparisons revealed marginally significant time differences between all three SM-Groups at p=0.07. The differences between Meditation and Control Group (Λ=0.65, F(11,39)=1.87, p=0.07) were reflected by the quartic trend-component (F(1,49)=5.40, p=0.02); see Fig. 31.11a.

Figure 31.11a   HR: SM-Groups' Tonic Response to Repetition of Warning at 215 s, N=75

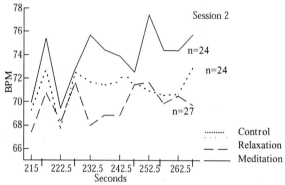

SM-Group X Time differences between Relaxers, Controls and Meditators

In contrast, the SM-Group X Time interaction for the same sequence of the first session was far away from any effect (Λ=0.60, F(11,62)=3.75, p=0.80) although the time values seemed to suggest one; see Fig. 31.11b.

Figure 31.11b, Heart Rate: Prospective SM-Groups' Tonic Response
to Repetition of Warning Stimulus at 215s, no differences, N=75

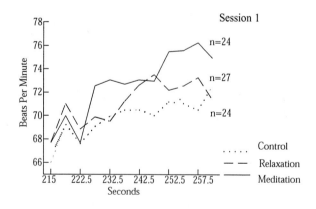

Session differences in Standard Error

There was no SM-Group X Time effect because of between SM-Group differences in variability in the first session (see Fig. 31.12a). Both Stress Management Groups had higher levels of variability than the Controls in the repetition sequence of session 1 and were diverse between each other in short latency as well as in the windows 227.5s respectively 237.5s - 247.5s.

Figure 31.12a, Heart Rate, prospective SM- Groups' Tonic Response
to Repetition of Warning, Standard Error of the Mean

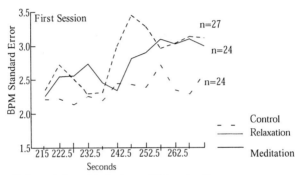

High variability in Meditation and Relaxation Group

The variability levels changed, however, in the second session. The variability of the trained Stress Management Groups was reduced in most of the windows compared to the variability change of the Controls. Only the last two windows at 12.5s and 7.5s before HI-Stimulus on-set were at a similar level of the Controls' variability (the last window at 262.5s was not calculated; see Fig. 31.12b).

Figure 31.12b, Heart Rate: SM-Groups' Tonic Response
to Repetition of Warning, Standard Error of the Mean

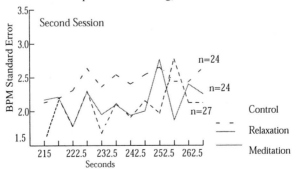

Lower variability for Meditators & Relaxers except 2 windows before HI-onset

The fact that responsivity varied less in those subjects who meditated or did muscle Relaxation for 4-5 weeks than in those who did not such practice suggests by itself some effect the methods had on the trainees.

3.1.3 Recovery from HI-Stimulus Impact for SM- Group

Goleman & Schwartz (1976) found greater stress recovery in experienced Meditators compared to Meditation beginners and Relaxers. They claimed that the experienced Meditators decelerated more post stimulation (relative to their pre-stimulus values) than the Control-beginners. Lehrer, Woolfolk et al. (1981,83) replicated this result with meditator beginners in comparison to Relaxers and waiting-list Controls. These studies did not employ a pre-training stress experiment and the subjects were tested only once after Stress Management training. In contrast, this study based on session comparison had to use multifactorial ANOVA on the pre- and post HI-stimulus minimum heart-rates of both sessions, which had shown greater habituation in the overall means with repetition for the Meditators compared to the Control subjects. Why not to check for a result in recovery as the authors from the seventies.

While those experimenters had used 15 seconds for sampling minimum heart-rate values pre and post stimulus we had to cover for the long latency period. Therefore we used the 5-sec-windows of the period 5-60 sec for post-stimulus and 60 sec for pre-stimulus onset. ANOVA was run on the four time-variables with SM-Group as between subject and Session and Time as within-subject factors. The results showed no effect at all: $F(2,66)= 0.51$, $p=0.79$ for between subject effect, $F(2,66) =0.01$, $p=0.99$ for SM-Group X Session X Time interaction $F(2,66)= 1.89$, $p=0.16$ for SM-Group X Session interaction. The near effect interaction of SM-Groups with the session overall mean occurred due to the elevated baseline value in the Meditation Group. Table 31.5 shows the Control Group with the tendency of greater deceleration scores sessions.

Table 31.5

Minimum Heart-Rate pre- and post- first HI-Stimulus, Deceleration Scores (Δ)

SM-GROUP		SESSION 1 HI-Stimulus 1			SESSION 2 HI-Stimulus 3		
		Pre	Post	Δ	Pre	Post	Δ
Meditation, SD	n=23	61.14 13.3	59.84 12.1	1.26	66.61 10.5	63.30 10.5	3.30
Relaxation, SD	n=25	61.60 11.4	61.60 14.0	0.0	61.80 7.7	58.86 7.4	2.94
Control, SD	n=23	60.57 10.9	58.09 11.2	2.47	63.09 10.5	58.26 10.8	4.83

3.1.4 Summary Heart Rate

In the first Session we found our hypotheses on individual differences in response to High Intensity stimulation confirmed. They were found in the response mean and its shape of both latencies post stimulus. In long latency there were tonic differences of Cardiac Subgroup over time reflected by differences in the quadratic and cubic trend components. In short latency we had differences over time between C.Subgroups also reflected by differences in the quadratic and cubic trend component.

However, no sufficient evidence was found for reflection of individual differences in the sequences post warning of an impending Stimulus of High Intensity. There was some evidence for sensitisation in the averaged means of the sequences post warning regarding the Accelerators. Since the differences in response to High Intensity Stimulation habituate within Session, the hypothesis on C.Subgroup specific effects of Stress Management could not be tested in the comparison of Sessions.

We found also some differences of prospective groups of Stress Management in the aggregated means of the warning sequences: The prospective Meditators were more responsive than the prospective Control Group (p=0.057).

The comparison of sessions had two main results: There was no dis-habituation of C.Subgroup differences in the period of long latency post High Intensity Stimulation and we had mainly a rejection of the hypothesis on activation reducing effects of Stress Management. However, the interaction effect of SM-Group with Session and Repetition showed that both positive Stress Management groups habituated in the second session's repetition phases to the Warning stimulus while the no-Stress Management-Controls sensitised with repetition of the Warning Stimulus in the second session. The Meditators' elevated resting baseline led to overall mean and Time differences with the two other SM-Groups in the first phasic Warning sequence.

The Meditators showed then a remarkable habituation to the Repetition of the Warning stimulus, which was reliably different from both other SM-Groups' responses within and between Session (Session X SM-Group X Repetition effect). The effect, however, had to be accounted for by an increment of resting baseline in the second session (regression to the mean) confirmed by the analysis of a smaller sample matched by baseline and gender, which showed no SM-Group differences. A similar SM-Group X Repetition effect was found in the High Intensity sequences of the second session but without Session being involved.

Differences between Stress Management methods were suggested by post-hoc analysis of reliable overall Time differences between SM-Groups in the tonic variables of warning (averaged means). This difference was a cumulative effect of differences between Meditators and Controls in the first session and Meditators and Relaxers in the second session's averaged means. In both post hoc comparisons the Meditators had higher heart rates than their competitors.

The hypothesis on Meditators' faster recovery post HI-stimulus impact could not be confirmed. A session comparison of both pre-post stimulus changes of minimum heart-rate had no effects into direction of hypothesis.

3.2 Blood Pressure

Introductory Comment

Systolic and diastolic blood-pressure were taken 3 times: The first measurement at laboratory arrival, the second about 30 minutes or so later after the subjects had filled in the questionnaires and were sitting in the experimental chair with electrodes attached to them. The third was taken after the experiment was over, with electrodes detached. Each measurement was taken twice with an interval of 3 minutes at the time and then averaged in order to reduce the error. So, we had the initial baseline, the resting or pre-experiment baseline and the post-experiment value (note: identical use of resting and pre-experiment baseline terms). Consequently, both baselines were analysed for changes before the main analysis of the pre-post experimental changes was run. The data-set for both sessions was not complete because in some cases at different time-points one of the measurement had been forgotten to be taken. For the comparison of sessions, complete 73 records were available for pre-post analyses and two less records were available for changes from Initial to Resting value. Both analyses were run with our between subject factors and Time and Session as within subject factors.

Systolic Bloodpressure

Initial baseline: There were no reliable differences in the between subject factors ($F_{(2,69)}=1.93$, p=0.15 for SM-Group, $F_{(1,69)}=0.07$, p=0.79 for C.Subgroup; $F_{(2,69)}=1.45$, p=0.24 for interaction.

Initial, Resting: There was a Time main effect ($F_{(1,65)}=24.39$, p<0.001; $\bar{X}_{Initial}=123.4$, $\bar{X}_{Resting}=119.2$mmHg) revealing a general "calming down" of resting baseline but the between subject factors were not involved in this event ($F_{(2,65)}=0.12$, p=0.89 for Time X SM-Group, $F_{(1,65)}=0.47$, p=0.50 for Time X C.Subgroup, $F_{(1,65)}=0.00$, p=1.00 for C.Subgroup; $F_{(2,65)}=0.65$, p=0.52 for SM-Group). There was no Session main effect ($F_{(1,65)}=0.62$, p=0.43) and again no interaction with the between-subject factors at mean level ($F_{(2,65)}=1.70$, p=0.19 for Session X SM-Group, $F_{(1,65)}=1.40$, p=0.24 for Session X C.Subgroup). There were no Session interaction effects at Time level either ($F_{(2,65)}=2.0$, p=0.15 for Session X Time X SM-Group, $F_{(1,65)}=0.12$, p=0.74 for Session X Time X C.Subgroup).

Resting (pre), post Experiment: Analysis of values showed no effects of the between subject factors ($F_{(2,70)}=0.65$, p=0.53 for SM-Group with one factor, $F_{(1,67)}=0.16$, p=0.69 for C.Subgroup, $F_{(2,67)}=1.03$, p=0.36 for between-subject factor interaction).

There was a Time effect ($F_{(1,67)}=4.50$, p=0.04) indicating within-subject changes There was no Session effect ($F_{(1,70)}=1.20$, p=0.29) but a marginal Session X SM-Group interaction ($F_{(2.70)}=2.50$, p=0.09). A significant difference between Meditation and Relaxation Group ($F_{(1,48)}=4.60$, p=0.04) was revealed by post-hoc test of hypothesis. While the Meditators namely had their overall mean increased from 118.3 mmHg in the first to 119.5 mmHg in the second session ($\Delta \bar{X}=1.25$mmHg) the Relaxation Group had a fall from 120.8 mmHg in the first to 116.9 mmHg in the second ($\Delta \bar{X} = -4.1$ mmHg)! The Control Group had lowered their session mean by 0.4mmHg (122.0-121.6). However, comparison with the Relaxers did not reach significance $(F(1,47)=1.93, p=0.17)$. Fig. 32.1a-b shows differences over Time insinuating multivariate analysis. However, this presentation was chosen for better clarity. It shows the linear differences between Relaxers and the other two groups. Only the Relaxers had a lower value post experiment than before experiment.

Figure 32.1a
Systolic BP: Prospective SM-Groups, three Measurements, Session 1

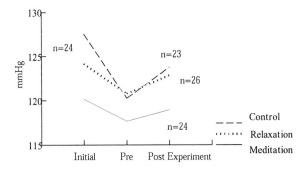

Figure 32.1b
Systolic BP: Stress Management Group, three Measurements, Session 2

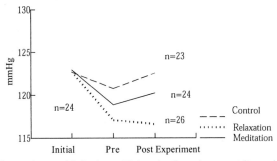

Differences between Meditation and Relaxation Group in pre-post Comparison

Diastolic Bloodpressure

*Initial Baseline:*There were overall mean differences of SM-Group $(F(2,68)=4.74, p=0.02,$ one factor); the Control subjects had higher levels at entering the laboratory than the Relaxation subjects ($\overline{X}$Control$=76.3$, $\overline{X}_{Relax}=68.7$mmHg, Tukey's test p<0.01). There was no reliable main effect of Session $(F(1,65)=2.81, p<0.10)$ but no interactions with the between subject factors $(F(2,65)=0.25, p=0.78$ for Session X SM-Group; $F(1,65)=0.35, p=0.56$ for Session X C.Subgroup, $F(1,65)=0.48, p=0.49$ for C.Subgroup effect).

Initial, Resting: There was a session main effect in initial to resting baseline (F(1,65)=3.90, p=0.05) because the overall mean of the second session was lowered. However, there was no interaction with SM-Group (F(2,65)=0.11, p=0.90). There was an all factor interaction of Session X Time X SM-Group X C.Subgroup instead (F(2,65)=3.93, p=0.02) hinting at C.Subgroup X SM-Group differences in the first session. Subsequent post-hoc tests found that in the first session the Accelerators of the Control Group had reliably different directional changes from Initial to Resting baseline (F(1,30)=8.03, p=0.02 for Control vs Meditation; F(1,30)=5.74, p<0.01 for Control vs Relaxation). While the Accelerators of both prospective SM- groups had gone down with their resting baselines, the Control-Accelerators had increased diastolic BP by 5.5 mmHg from entering the laboratory until start of the experiment. The values can be read from Table 32.1

Table 32.1 Diastolic BP: First Session for Accelerators in SM-Groups Baseline Group Means with Standard Error

Accelerators in prospective SM-Groups	Initial Baseline		Resting Baseline	
Meditation	72.5	3.1	70.4	3.2
Relaxation	71.2	3.2	67.8	3.4
Control	73.7	3.5	79.1	3.7

Figure 32.2a-b

Diastolic BP: Prosp. Stress Management Groups, First Session

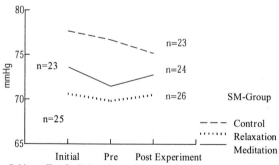

Between Subject effect for Relaxation and Control Group in pre-post Comparison

In the second session the Accelerators of the Control Group had reduced their increase from initial to resting (Δ+5.5 to Δ+1.4mmHg) while the Accelerators of the Relaxation Group had increased from Δ-3.4 to Δ+1.5mmHg; see session differences from Initial to Resting for SM-Group in Fig. 32.1a,b). Pre/post-experiment: There was an overall mean effect of SM-Group in the diastolic time-variables (F(2,70)=3.11, p=0.05, with SM-Group alone) which was confirmed by Tukey's Test with overall mean differences between Relaxation ($\overline{X}$=68.8mmHg) and Control Group ($\overline{X}$=75.3mmHg; p<0.02). There was a main effect of Session (F(1,70)= 5.95, p=0.02) but no interaction with SM-Group (F(2,70)=0.17, p=0.84; F(1,67)=0.24, p=0.62 for C.Subgroup effect). See the differences for initial, resting and post experiment for both sessions in Fig.32.2a-b.

Figure 32.2b

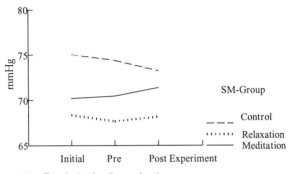

Diastolic BP: Stress Management Groups, Second Session

No effects in Session Comparison!

Summary

The diastolic time-point variables of the first session were quite biased by selection. The Control Group had a higher level throughout, which was mirrored in reliable differences between Control and Relaxation Group of initial baseline and in the overall mean of pre- and post experiment value. Furthermore: Accelerators from the Control Group showed a different pattern than the Accelerators of the other two SM-Groups and from the non-Accelerators: Starting from the 73.7 mmHg initial DBP, they increased their pre-experimental baseline to 79.1 mmHg. That explained the different, vertex-free shape of the Control Group's time-line in the first session's graphic display (Fig. 32.2a,b).

The systolic variables were not reliably biased. There were some initial mean differences between Meditators and Controls though (Fig. 32.1a). However, the Session X SM-Group mean differences of pre-post experiment measurement can be appreciated ignoring these initial differences because the Resting Baselines were similar between Relaxers and Meditators. There were reliable session differences between both practising Stress Management groups: While the Meditators had increased their low level of Systolic BP by 1.2mmHg (118.3-119.5mmHg) the Relaxers had come down from almost 121 mmHg to below 117 mmHg overall mean of pre /post experiment SBP. The Controls had only a 0.4 mmHg difference (p=0.17). Thus, the differences occurred more due to a reduction in the Relaxation subjects' response mean than to an increase of the Meditators' response mean.

3.3 Respiration-Rate

Introductory Comment

We measured the frequency of complete and incomplete inhalation/exhalation cycles by frequency per minute (cpm). The incomplete cycles were counted by 25% of the whole cycle and the measurement of the cycles in the sequences post-stimulation started with stimulus on-set. Consequently each sequence consisted only of one time-variable quite in contrast to the other variables read from the polygraph. The resting baselines as reference points for the first warning periods were taken from the last three minutes of the five minutes resting period before the first warning stimulus. The recovery baselines as reference points for the repetition-warning sequence were taken from the second minute post High Intensity-stimulus. Since the HI-sequences had been related to the previous Warning sequence before (last 5-sec-value), the pre-HI- stimulus baselines were identical with the values of the previous warning sequence.

Again, a comparison of both sessions was run in order to look for parallel effects of the Cardiac Subgroup factor and for a selection bias reflected in interactions with the Stress Management Group factor. This would allow us to control for somatic coupling with events in Heart Rate.

Resting/Recovery Baselines (N=73) and Sequences post Warning (N=72)

Resting and recovery: The first session's resting baselines were not reliably different in the between subject factors ($F_{(2,67)}=0.36$, $p=0.70$ for SM-Group, $F_{(1,67)}=1.69$, $p=0.20$ for C.Subgroup and $F_{(2,67)}=1.48$, $p=0.24$ for interaction).

Session comparison of all four baselines did not reveal any effect of the between subject factors ($F_{(2,66)}=0.56$, $p=0.58$ for SM-Group, $F_{(1,66)}=0.52$, $p=0.48$ for C.Subgroup and $F_{(2,66)}=0.92$, $p=0.40$ for interaction). There was no session effect ($F_{(1,66)}=0.12$, $p=0.73$) and no interaction with the between subject factors ($F_{(2,66)}=0.12$, $p=0.82$ for Session X SM-Group and $F_{(1,66)}=0.95$, $p=0.33$ for Session X C.Subgroup). There was no repetition effect either ($F_{(1,66)}=2.15$, $p=0.15$) but an interaction effect was there of SM-Group X C.Subgroup X Repetition ($F_{(2,66)}=3.46$, $p=0.04$). This interaction did not involve Session ($F_{(2,66)}=0.32$, $p=0.73$), however, the main variance for this effect was found in the first session's baselines between the Accelerators of Meditation and Control Group ($F_{(1,41)}=9.80$, $p=0.003$). The Meditation-Accelerators had increased their respiration rate by 0.75 cycles in the recovery baseline, their counterpart of the Control Group had clearly habituated by reducing their rate by 1.26 cycles.

Warning sequences: As explained the minute values of the warning sequences served as baselines to the HI-stimulus sequences, therefore they are reported here. There was no effect at overall mean level for any of the between-subject factors in the warning sequences ($F_{(1,66)}=0.30$, $p=0.59$ for C.Subgroup; $F_{(2,66)}=0.68$, $p=0.51$ for SM-Group; $F_{(2,66)}=1.06$, $p=0.35$ for interaction). There were no effects of the within-subject factors ($F_{(1,66)}=0.75$, $p=0.39$ for Session; $F_{(1,66)}=1.58$, $p=0.21$ for Repetition, $F_{(1,66)}=3.17$, $p=0.08$ for Time) and no interaction effect of Session with any of the between-subject factors ($F_{(1,66)}=0.45$, p=0.51 for C.Subgroup; F(2,66)=0.61, p=0.55 for SM-Group, F(2,66)=0.19, p=0.83 for all-factor-interaction).

Sequences post High Intensity (N=71)

Again there were no main effects of the between-subject factors (F(1,65)=0.25, p=0.62 for C.Subgroup,   F(2,65)=0. 46, p=0.63 for SM-Group, F(2,65)=0.89, p=0.42 for interaction). The within subject factors had no reliable effects on the time variables either (F(1,65)=0.17, p=0.68 for Session, F(1,65)=2.18, p=00.15 for Repetition, F(1,65)=1.86, p=0.18 for Time).

However, the between-subject factors interacted with the within-subject factors at mean level: There was a Session X Repetition X SM-Group interaction effect (F(2,68)=5.35, p<0.01) and post-hoc test of hypothesis showed significant differences between Meditators and both Controls (F(1,42)=7.41, p<0.01) and Relaxers (F(1,47)=7.92, p<0.01) over Session X Repetition. In the second session, the Meditators reversed their direction of change from first stimulation to repetition. While they sensitised in the first session, they habituated in the second, see Fig. 33.1.

. Figure 33.1

Respiration Rate: Session X Repetition X SM-Group interaction effect between Meditators and the two other SM-Groups

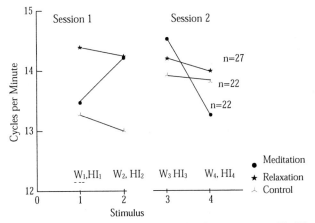

Each value represents the averaged mean of Warning and High Intensity sequence. The Warning mean was used as baseline for High Intensity mean. Cycles were counted by 25% ratios.

The averaged values of Warning and HI-stimulus sequence means showed that the Meditators had increased their rate by 0.74 cpm in the first session while the controls and Relaxers had theirs reduced by -0.27 and -0.15 cpm respectively. In the second session the Meditators reduced their rate by -1.27 cpm while the other Groups had only minor reductions by -0.11cpm and -0.21cpm. These values were the basis for the significant differences at p<0.01.

All SM-Groups had raised their breathing rate in the second session and the Meditators' major reduction with repetition can therefore not entirely be attributed to the regression of the mean rule.

On the other hand: The meditators' first Warning sequence-mean did contribute to the variance for the effect described above as can be seen in Fig. 33.2-3 with all values along the time scale. The HI-values are encircled for better comprehension.

Figure 33.2

Respiration-Rate: Resting/ Recovery baselines and sequences post Warning and HI-Stimulus with repetition for Stress-Management Groups, N=71

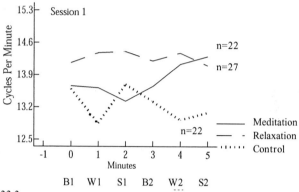

Figure 33.3

Respiration-Rate: Resting/ Recovery Baseline, Warning and HI-Stimulus Sequences with Repetition for SM- Group, N=71

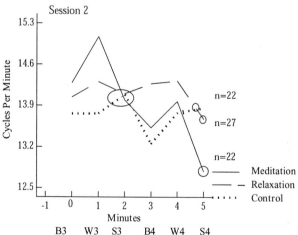

Each value equals the average mean per sequence, W used as baseline for HI.

There was another Session X Time interaction but for the C.Subgroup factor (F(1,69)=6.25, p<0.02 for C.Subgroup X Session X Repetition X Time, with one factor). Analysis of first session's time variables revealed a 3-way interaction of C.Subgroup with Repetition and Time (F(1,69)=7.43, p<0.01). A C.Subgroup X Time interaction effect was found in the repetition sequence of HI- stimulus (F(1,69)=4.82, p=0.03). The Accelerators had a lower respiration rate ($\Delta \overline{X}_{ACCEL}$= 0.59) than their counterpart who breathed more frequently ($\Delta \overline{X}_{NONACC}$ =-0.48) compared to their baseline-Warning sequence (Fig. 33.4; W2 and S2 on the time scale). The effect occurred due to different tendencies of the Cardiac Subgroups during the first session, see Fig. 33.4-5 followed by more explanation.

Figure 33.4

Respiration Rate: C.Subgroup X Session X Repetition X Time effect, Average mean per sequence, Warning used as baseline for HI-S sequence

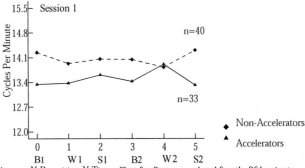

C.Subgroup X Repetition X Time effect for first, second and fourth, fifth minute

Figure 33.5

Respiration Rate: C.Subgroup X Session X Repetition X Time effect (cont.), Average mean per sequence, Warning used as baseline for HI- Sequence

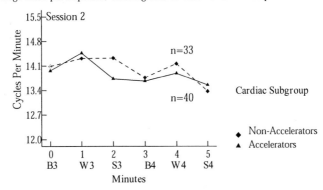

While the Accelerators breathed at a lower rate than their counterpart during the first part of session 1, they increased their rate in the repetition-of-warning-sequence from which they had to come down to their normal baseline level. The non-Accelerators, in

contrast, had to increase their rate in order to reach baseline level. The C.Subgroup differences were abolished in the second session (Fig. 33.5) because the Accelerators had increased their resting and recovery baseline rate to the level of their counterpart. However, this session-baseline shift was not significant as has been reported in the baseline paragraph (Session X C.Subgroup p=0.33).

Summary Respiration Rate

There were no reliable differences in the respiration baseline values of SM-Group and Cardiac Subgroup. There were no effects in the warning sequences but there were SM-Group differences over Session and Repetition in the sequences post HI-Stimulus, which was based on averaged Warning and HI-Stimulus sequences (because the Warning mean constituted the baseline value for HI-Stimulus sequence mean). The Meditators had an increase to the first HI-stimulus of the second Session and showed faster habituation with repetition of HI-stimulus. The habituation value was below their resting baseline of the first Session.

Analysis also showed different tendencies for Accelerators of Meditation and Control Group: the former tended to sensitise in recovery baseline, the latter to habituate.

3.4 Muscle Activity, - Electromyogram -

Introductory Comment

The data from the electromyographic recordings contained two response measures: the levels of muscle activity during the sequences post stimulation and the direct responses to the stimuli during stimulation. The involuntary contraction of the neck-muscles at the time-point of stimulation represents what is known in the literature as the startle-reflex (Graham 1975).

So, three measures were taken from the data: the direct response to the (two kinds of) stimuli (startle), the baseline and the level of activity during the rest of each post-stimulation sequence both regarded as tonic measures. Baselines were taken from the resting levels at least 10 seconds before moderate stimulation (Resting and Recovery) and from the last 5-second window before High-Intensity Stimulation. The change-scores from baseline of the response-peak drawn by the polygraph during stimulation were counted as startle. That was one value for the warning stimulus and two values for the HI-double stimulus interleaved by a second (Methods). The levels of tonic electro-myographic activity were read from eleven 5-sec-windows starting with 5 seconds post stimulus onset.

As for the previous sections the session-comparison of 67 complete records was dedicated to the search of differences in the between-subject factors and in their interactions with the within-subject factors, primarily Session but also Repetition and Time. Differences of Cardiac C.Subgroup linked to the Session factor could suggest reflections of the CDR during Session I. Differences of Stress Management Group linked to Session could suggest either differences due to non-random allocation (Session 1) or following training (Session 2). However, also overall differences of the mean or over time would indeed suggest a selection bias. Interactions of the between-subject factor also could suggest both: effects of training or a selection bias. Therefore, an analysis of the first session was likely to follow the comparison.

Baselines (B1-B4, W1 (12) - W4 (12))

There were no effects of the single grouping factors on the overall mean of Resting/Recovery and pre-HI-stimulus baselines (all F<1). However, there was an interaction effect in Resting/Recovery ($F(2,61)= 3.46$, p=0.04) and a marginal one in pre-HI-stimulus baselines ($F(2,61)=0.26$, p=2.88, p=0.06). Post-hoc test showed reliable C.Subgroup differences within the Relaxation Group (p=0.01, for Control Group p=0.4) but only for the baselines of Session I. Further testing of the first session's Resting/Recovery baseline-mean showed reliable C.Subgroup differences into direction of hypothesis for the Relaxation Group ($\overline{X}ACC=40.3\mu v$, $\overline{X}NACC=14.3\mu v$; Control Group: $\overline{X}ACC=15.2\mu v$, $\overline{X}NACC=29.3\mu v$). The C.Subgroup-differences in the Meditation Group also were into direction of hypothesis but were not significant.

At within-level there was no effect of Session in any of the baselines ($F(1,62)=0.04$, p=0.84 for pre-HI-stimulus) nor of Repetition ($F(1,61)=2.10$, p=0.15 for Resting/Recovery $F(1,61)=0.38$, p=0.31 for pre HI-stimulus). There were no interactions with the between-subject factors (F(1,61)=0.85 for Session X C.Subgroup; F(2,61)=0.01, p=1.0 for Session X SM-Group; F(2,61)=0.08, p=0.92 for Session X C.Subgroup X SM-Group).

Sequences post Warning

Tonic Response (B1-B4, W1(2-12) -W4(2-12))

There was nothing like an effect for the single between-subject factors (F(1,61)=0.58, p=0.45 for C.Subgroup, F(2,61)=0.23, p=0.80 for SM-Group). Yet again there was an interaction effect of C.Subgroup X SM-Group (F(2,61=3.46, p=0.04) suggesting continuation of the C.Subgroup differences found in the Resting/Recovery baselines of the Relaxation Group.

At within level there was no effect of Session (F(1,61)=0.04, p=0.84) or Time (Λ=0.86 F(11,51)=0.78, p=0.66) though Repetition came close to an effect (F(1,61)=2.47, p=0.12) and the heightened values of the repetition sequences suggested a sensitising tendency.

There was no interaction of the within and between subject factors suggesting no differences of first session in the factors (Λ=0.93, F(11,51)=0.37, p=0.37 for C.Subgroup X Time; F(1,61)=0.78, p=0.38 for Session X C.Subgroup; Λ=0.68, F(22,102)=0.97, p=0.51 for SM-Group X Time, F(2,61)=0.00, p=1.00 for Session X SM-Group). Finally there was no effect for C.Subgroup X SM-Group X Time interaction (Λ=0.72, F(22,102)=0.82, p=0.70) suggesting that the baseline differences of the between-subject factor interaction were not maintained over time. Considering the lack of effects in the interactions of the between subject factors the original hypothesis (Session X Repetition X Time X C.Subgroup X SM-Group) needed not to be tested.

Startle (ChScW1(1) - ChScW4(1))

The four change-score values were tested with the two between subject factors and Session and Repetition as within subject factors. There was no effect of the between subject factors (F(1,61)=0.53, p=0.47 for C.Subgroup; F(2,61)=1.63, p=0.20 for SM-Group; F(2,61)=0.84, p=0.44 for interaction).

There was no Session main effect (F(1,61)=1.10, p=0.30) but a strong effect of Repetition was there (F(1,61)=24.38, p<0.001, ΔREP =32.4µv) because of habituation. There was no interaction of Session with SM-Group (F(2,61)=1.21, p=0.30) but there were two interactions with C.Subgroup that could not be ignored due to the hypothesis on individual differences: A marginally reliable C.Subgroup X Session effect was there (F(1,61)=3.40, p=0.07) and a near interaction effect of C.Subgroup X Session X Repetition (F(1,61)=2.66, p=0.11). The Cardiac Subgroups showed a reverse pattern in both sessions: In the first session the Accelerators had a lower session-mean in startle ($\overline{X}$ACCEL=35.0µv) than the non-Accelerators ($\overline{X}$NonACC=46.5µv) but they doubled their mean in the second session ($\overline{X}$ACCEL=69.9µv) in contrast to their habituating counterpart ($\overline{X}$NonACC= 37.0µv).

Figure 34.1   EMG: Cardiac Subgroups' Startle post Warning and Repetition,
Session X C.Subgroup effect: p<0.07, N=67

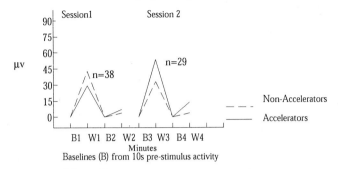

Sequences post High Intensity

Tonic (W1(12) - W4 (12), HI-S1(3-13) – HI-S 4(3-13))

The between-subject factors had no effects on the overall mean: $F(1,61)=0.83$, $p=0.37$ for C.Subgroup and $F(2,61)=0.16$, $p=0.85$ for SM-Group. There were no main effects of Session ($F(1,61)=0.05$, $p=0.83$), Repetition ($F(1.61)=0.54$, $p=0.47$) or Time ($\Lambda = 0.79$, $F(11,51)=1.21$, $p<0.30$) either. Unsurprisingly then there was nothing for the hypotheses, interactions of the between-subject factors with session: Session X Time X C.Subgroup ($\Lambda=0.77$, $F(11,51)=1.38$, $p=0.21$; Session X Time X SM-Group ($\Lambda=0.70$, $F(22,102)=0.89$, $p=0.60$). Overall interactions of the between-subject factors with Time did not suggest any interactions in the first session's values either (all $F<1$). Thus, there was no reflection of the CDR in the tonic response levels to HI-stimulus.

Startle (ChSc HI-S1(1-2) – ChScHI-S4(1-2))

ANOVA of the 2 x 4 change-scores revealed neither main effects of SM-Group ($F(2,61)=0.04$, $p=0.96$) or C.Subgroup ($F(1,61)=1.85$, $p=0.18$) nor an interaction of the two ($F(2,61)=0.28$, $p=0.76$).

However, it revealed effects of all the within subject factors {$F(1,61)=6.44$, $p=0.01$ for Session; ($\overline{X}$SESSION1=108.5µv, $\overline{X}$SESSION2=78.6µv) $F(1,61)=37.63$ $p<0.001$ for Repetition (Δ $\overline{X}$REP=213.0µv) and $F(1,61)=120.60$, $p<0.001$ for Time ($\Delta=131.2$µv)}. Both, Session and Repetition effect suggested habituation to repeated presentation of HI-stimulus and so did the Time effect for the habituation within double-stimulus. Due to habituation there were multiple interactions between them. Session X Repetition: $F(1,61)=8.85$, $p<0.01$ (ΔSES1=256.7µv, ΔSES2=116.9µv), Session X Repetition X Time: $F(1,61)=5.08$, $p=0.03$ and Session X Time: $F(1,61)=4.61$, $p=0.04$.

The SM-Group factor interacted with all the within subject factors though not to effect size (Session X Repetition X Time X SM-Group: $F(2,61)=1.99$, $p=0.15$). To look for a trend in this important variable a post-hoc test of hypothesis was applied to the data. There was indeed an effect in the second session (F(2,64)=3.34, p=0.04) with differences between Relaxation and Meditation Group (F(1,44)=7.02, p=0.01).

The Meditators did not habituate to repetition of HI-stimulus (S4) as they did in the first session and indeed in other variables, and as the Relaxers did here in both sessions. The Relaxers also habituated faster within the double-stimulus S3 (Fig 34.2) which was expressed by the involvement of the Time factor. For better clarity, only the two different SM-Groups are shown in the display. The values of the Control subjects have thought to be positioned between Relaxers and Meditators.

Figure 34.2   EMG: SM-Groups' Startle post HI-Stimulus with Repetition, 2 Change Scores post onset, faster habituating Relaxation Group in second Session

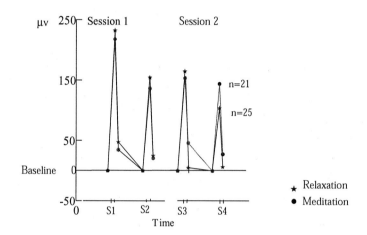

Summary

There were some initial differences in the first session's tonic analysis. The Relaxation Group showed C.Subgroup differences in their tonic data regarding both Resting and Recovery baselines of the first session. There was also a continuation of this effect in the first Warning overall mean, but nothing of the kind over Time. There were no effects regarding the main hypothesis whatsoever.

Startle analysis of the Warning-sequences showed a reverse session effect in the C.Subgroup factor with differences in the second session due to habituation of the Non-Accelerators and sensitisation of the Accelerators. In High Intensity sequences there was a trend of faster habituation for the Relaxers in comparison to the Meditators but not to the Controls. In fact, the Meditators showed a tendency to sensitise with repetition in the second session compared to the first session and to the Relaxers.

3.5 Skin Conductance

Baselines

There were interaction effects between SM-Group and C.Subgroup in the overall means of both, resting/recovery $(F(2,60)=3.29,$ p=0.04) and pre-HI-stimulus baselines $(F(2,60)=4.34,$ p=0.02). Both effects interacted further with Session $(F(2,60)=4.69,$ p=0.01 for pre-warning, $F(2,60)=4.26,$ p=0.02 for pre-HI-Stimulus). Interactions between C.Subgroup and SM-Group were found in the baseline variables of the first session $(F(2,63)=8.14,$ p=0.001 for pre-Warning; $F(2,63)=9.07,$ p<0.001 for pre-HI-Stimulus). Post-hoc tests of hypotheses revealed C.Subgroup differences in Meditation and Control Group (Table 35.1-2).

Table 35.1	Resting/ Recovery Baselines, SM-Group X C.Subgroup, Post-Hoc Test			
SM-GROUP C.Subgroup	B1 (RESTING)	B2 (RECOVERY)	$\overline{X}$ SESSION1	P<
MEDITATION				
Accelerators	0.846	0.950	0.898	0.01
non-Accelerators	1.104	1.212	1.16	
RELAXATION				
Accelerators	1.009	1.112	1.06	
non-Accelerators	0.963	1.080	1.02	
CONTROL				
Accelerators	1.246	1.271	1.26	0.01
non-Accelerators.	0.981	1.033	1.01	

Table 35.2	Baselines, Pre-HI-Stimulus SM-Group X C.Subgroup, Post-Hoc Test			
SM-GROUP C.Subgroup	**W1$_{(12)}$**	**W2$_{(12)}$**	**$\overline{X}_{SESSION1}$**	**P<**
MEDITATION				
Accelerators	0.926	1.006	0.97	0.01
non-Accelerators.	1.167	1.274	1.22	
RELAXATION				
Accelerators	1.092	1.148	1.12	
non-Accelerators	1.076	1.104	1.09	
CONTROL				
Accelerators	1.282	1.317	1.30	0.01
non-Accelerators.	1.009	1.046	1.03	

The C.Subgroup differences in the SM-Groups were not consistent in their direction. The Accelerators of the Meditation Group were well below the level of their counter-part in stark contrast to the direction of differences in the Control Group and Relaxation Group. The effect of self-selection in the baselines had several other effects in its trail for both kinds of post-stimulus sequences as will be reported further below.

There were no other effects in the baseline variables: Pre-Warning: $F(1,60)=0.05$, $p=0.82$ for Session; $F(1,60)=0.39$, $p=0.54$ for C.Subgroup; $F(2,60)=0.56$, $p=0.58$ for SM-Group; $F(1,60)=0.68$, $p=0.41$ for Session X C.Subgroup. Pre-HI-Stimulus: $F(1,60)=0.51$, $p=0.48$ for Session; $F(1,60)=1.09$, $p=0.30$ for C.Subgroup; $F(2,60)=0.39$, $p=0.68$ for SM-Group; $F(1,60)=1.26$, $p=0.27$ for Session X C.Subgroup; $F(2,60)=0.30$, $p=0.74$ for Session X SM-Group.

Sequences post Warning (B1, W1-4$_{(1-11)}$)

Between and within-subject main effects: There were no effects of SM-Group (F(2,60)=0.42, p=0.66) or C.Subgroup (F(1,64)=0.49, p=0.49) in the overall mean. At within subject level there were main effects of Repetition (F(1,60)=17.84, p<0.001) and Time (Λ=0.23, F(11,54)=16.31, p<0.001) but none of Session (F(1,64)=0.55, p=0.46). The Repetition effect related to increased values in the second warning sequence suggesting sensitisation ($\Delta_{REPETITION}$ =0.051 logSC).

Interactions of C.Subgroup: There was a marginal interaction effect for Session X Repetition X Time X C.Subgroup (Λ=0.73, F(11,54)=1.78, p=0.08, for one factor) accompanied by a quadratic component of similar size (F(1,64)=3.26, p=0.07) and for Session X Time X C.Subgroup (Λ=0.74, F(11,54)=1.70, p=0.098).

The means of C.Subgroup- and a tendency of differences in the quadratic trend (p=0.07) overall were suggesting effects in the period of short latency covered by the first three 5-second-windows. Therefore the response in the first 13 seconds post onset reflected by the first three 5-sec-windows at 2.5 sec, 7.5 sec, 12.5 sec (W1-4$_{(1-3)}$) in relation to the baseline (B1-4) was analysed with C.Subgroup, Session, Repetition and Time. In fact there was a Session X Repetition X Time X C.Subgroup effect (Λ=0.86, F(3,62)=3.33, p<0.03) and a Time X C.Subgroup effect (Λ=0.86, F(3,62)=3.51, p=0.02; Time effect: Λ=0.28, F(3,62)=52.52, p<0.001). Again there was neither a main effect of C.Subgroup (F(1,64)=0.33, p=0.57) nor of Session (F(1,64)=0.42, p=0.52).

The analysis of the first three 5-sec-windows of the second session's first sequence showed reliable C.Subgroup differences at Time level (Λ=0.81, F(3,63)=4.80, p<0.01 for C.Subgroup X Time) reflected by a linear (F(1,65)=4.93, p=0.03) and a cubic trend-component (F(1,65)=14.63, p,0.001). The Accelerators showed a steeper slope than their counterparts from the 2.5-sec-window to the 7.5-sec-window and consequently a smaller cubic component in the three windows post on-set, see Fig. 32.2c. There were no C.Subgroup X Time differences in the repetition sequence (Λ=0.95, F(3,63)=1.05, p=0.38, Fig. 32.2d). In the first session, in contrast, we had no Time differences in the first (Fig. 32.2a) and marginal differences in the repetition-sequence (Fig. 32.2b).

Figure 35.2a
SCL: Cardiac Subgroups' Phasic Response to first Warning (W1), Onset at Zero

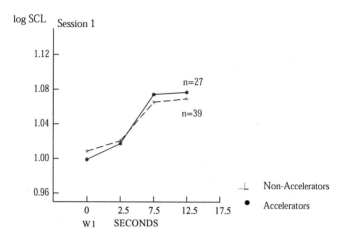

Figure 35.2b SCL: Cardiac Subgroups' Phasic Response to
Repetition of Warning, Recovery Baseline Shift Overall

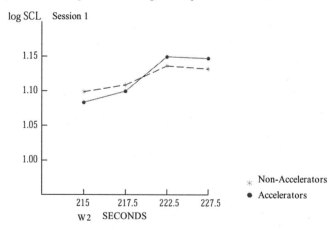

There was no reliable all-factor-interaction effect ($\Lambda=0.61$, $F(22,100)=1.29$, $p<0.20$ for Session X Repetition X Time X C.Subgroup X SM-Group), nevertheless, the increased levels of the Meditation-Accelerators suggested influence on the 4-way interaction effect analysed in the previous paragraph and which is shown in the graphic display of Figures 35.2a-d.

Figure 35.2c

    SCL: Cardiac Subgroups' Phasic response to first warning, W3,
    C.Subgroup X Time effect, reflected by linear and cubic trend-component

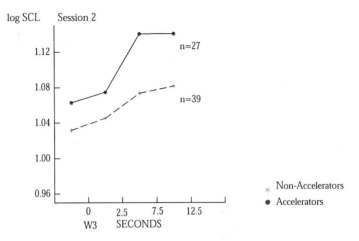

Figure 35.2d

    SCL: Cardiac Subgroups' Phasic response to Repetition of Warning (W4)
    No differences

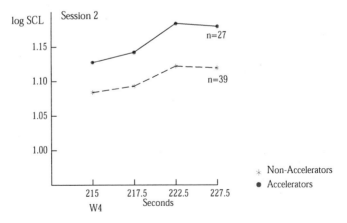

Interactions of SM-Group: There was a Session X Time X SM-Group interaction effect ($\Lambda=0.52$, $F(22,10)=1.79$, $p=0.03$), which could not be found in the second session (Time X SM-Group $\Lambda=0.69$, $F(22,108)=1.00$, $p=0.46$). There was only a "near effect" in the time-variables of the first session in the multivariate statistics ($\Lambda=0.63$, $F(22,112)=1.33$, $p=0.17$ for SM-Group X Time; Time main effect: $\Lambda=0.27$, $F(11,56)=13.67$, $p<0.001$). Clearly, there had not been any reliable differences between the SM-Groups in the time variables of the first session. However, because the Session factor had been involved in the grand analysis the interaction is pictured in the display of Fig. 35.1 and shows mild SM-Group differences in the period of long latency.

Figure 35.1 SCL : SM-Groups' Tonic Response to first session's warnings, Averaged Means, 11 Five-Sec-Windows (2.5s – 57.5s post onset)

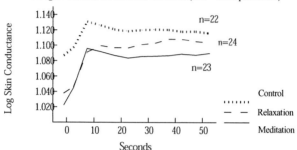

Interactions Between Subject factors: As in the Baselines there was an interaction effect of both SM-Group and C.Subgroup in the overall mean ($F(2,60)=3.911$, $p<0.03$) that further interacted with Session ($F(2,60)=4.40$, $p=0.02$ for Session X SM-Group X C.Subgroup). Post-hoc test showed a C.Subgroup X Session effect in the Meditation Group ($F(1,19)=9.00$, $p=0.01$) because the Accelerators had increased their levels in the second session ($\bar{X}_{ACCMED}=0.197$, $\bar{X}_{NACCMED}=-0.071$) as a consequence of the baseline shift analysed further above. The session differences of the Cardiac Subgroups in the three Stress Management Groups are shown in the graphic display of Fig 35.3.

Sequences post High - Intensity Stimulus

Again there were factor interactions in the overall mean: ($F(2,60)=4.87$, $p=0.01$ for Session X SM-Group X C.Subgroup: $F(2,60)=3.95$, $p=0.02$ for SM-Group X C.Subgroup). Again the Session X C.Subgroup differences occurred in the Meditation Group (see Fig. 35.4 overleaf).

The between subject factor interaction effects in the two stimulus type sequences presumably happened due to non-random allocation to SM. There was no effect of the between subject factors on the overall mean $F(2,60)=0.37$, $p=0.70$ for SM-Group, $F(1,60)=1.26$, $p=0.27$ for C.Subgroup. There was a main effect of Time ($\Lambda=0.27$, $F(11,50)=12.27$, $p<0.001$) but none of Session ($F(1,60)=0.00$, $p=0.99$) and there was no interaction effect of the between subject factors with one of the within-subject factors ($\Lambda=0.65$, $F(22,100)=1.09$, $p=0.37$ for Session X Repetition X Time X SM-Group,: $\Lambda=0.81$, $F(11,50)=1.06$, $p=0.41$ for C.Subgroup X Session X Repetition X Time).

Results, Skin Conductance Level -SCL

Fig. 35.3 LogSCL, Tonic Response to Warnings aggregated, C.Subgroup in SM-Group

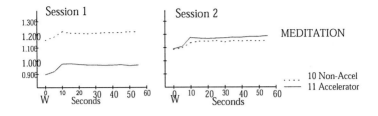

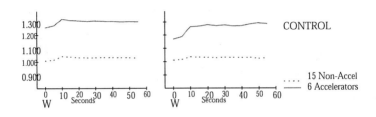

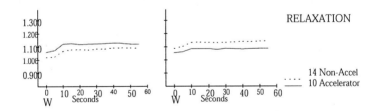

Figure 35.4
LogSCL: Tonic Response to HI-Stimulus with Repetition, averaged, C.Subgroups in SM-Groups

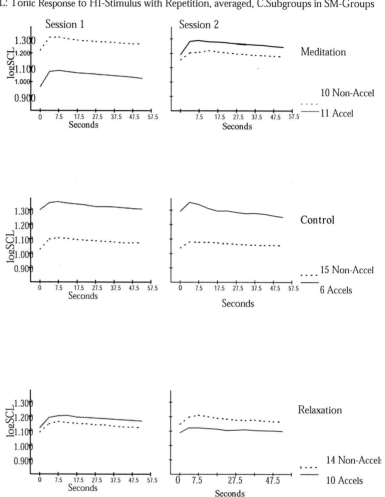

Summary

We had a selection bias based interaction effect of the between subject factors in the baselines of resting and recovery, before warning that is: there were C.Subgroup differences in both Control and Meditation Group but not in the Relaxation Group. However, these differences were not consistent in direction: whilst the baselines of the Control-Accelerators were typically higher than those of the Control-Non-Accelerators, the

Meditation C.Subgroups showed the expected pattern of Accelerators being higher than their counterparts.

These initial between-Group differences of C.Subgroup were the basis for session-effects (Session X SM-Group X C.Subgroup) in the overall mean of both Warning and HI-sequences because the differences within Meditation-Group were abolished in the second session. The Accelerators (Meditation) had increased their levels almost to the first session levels of the non-Accelerators and those had reduced their levels in the meantime. The differences within the Control Group had remained much the same.

There was a third session effect involving repetition in parallel to the results in phasic heart rate (Session X Repetition X Time X C.Subgroup). Reliable C.Subgroup differences over time reflected by differences in response shape appeared in the first three 5-sec-windows (13s post stimulus) of the second session's first warning-sequence. Those "accelerations" did not sensitise however, they vanished with repetition of Warning.

3.6 Subjective Measures - HI-Stimulus, Anxiety, Mood

3.6.1 Ratings of HI-Stimulus (N=74)

The analysis of the ratings with SM-Group and C.Subgroup as between subject factors and Session as within-subject factor did not reveal any differences:

Loudness: $F_{(2.68)}=0.68$, $p=0.51$ for SM-Group; $F_{(1,68)}=0.25$, $p=0.62$ for C.Subgroup, $F_{(2,68)}=0.54$, $p=0.58$ for interaction and $F_{(2,68)}=0.12$, $p=0.89$ for C.Subgroup X SM-Group X Session. There was no Session effect ($F_{(1,68)}=2.15$, $p<0.15$) and no effect for Session X SM-Group ($F_{(2,71)}=1.93$, $p=0.15$ for one factor). The means for SM-Groups (Table and Figure 36.1) showed different directional changes for the Meditators compared to the other Groups. They attributed relatively more loudness to the HI-stimulus in the second session while the others, in particular the Relaxers, did less so (Fig. 36.1). There was no interaction effect for Session X C.Subgroup ($F_{(1,68)}=0.49$, $p=0.49$, see Table 36.2 for C.Subgroup values.

Table 36.1:   **LOUDNESS of HI-Stimulus, SM-Group, Means, SE**

Session	Meditation		Relaxation		Control	
First	4.69	0.28	4.81	0.25	4.39	0.35
Second	4.78	0.28	4.28	0.26	4.21	0.30

Figure 36.1

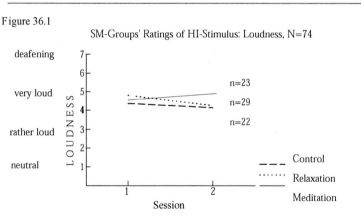

SM-Groups' Ratings of HI-Stimulus: Loudness, N=74

Table 36.2 LOUDNESS of HI-Stimulus, Cardiac Subgroup, Means, SE

Session	Accelerators		Non-Accelerators	
First	4.68	0.24	4.61	0.20
Second	4.55	0.24	4.26	0.21

Unpleasantness: There was no effect either in this variable (F(2,71)=0.66, p=0.52 for SM-Group; F(1,72)=1.45, p=0.23 for C.Subgroup and F(2,68)=0.74, p=0.48 for SM-Group X C.Subgroup and F(2,68)=1.58, p=0.21 for 3-way interaction with Session). There was again no Session effect (F(2,68)=2.46, p=0.12) and there was neither an interaction with SM-Group (F(2,71)=0.98, p=0.38) nor with C.Subgroup (F(1,72)=0.57, p=0.45). See Tables 36.3-4 and Figure 36.2.

Table 36.3   UNPLEASANTNESS of HI- Stimulus, SM-Group, Means & SE

Session	Meditation		Relaxation		Control	
First	4.65	0.33	4.65	0.30	4.49	0.35
Second	4.65	0.28	4.04	0.26	4.25	0.30

Tables and Figures for SM-Group show that the Meditators had relatively higher levels of ratings and remained unchanged in the second session. The Controls also remained unchanged but the Relaxers tended to rate the HI-stimulus lower in the second session.

Figure 36.2

SM-Groups' Ratings of HI-Stimulus: Unpleasantness, N=74

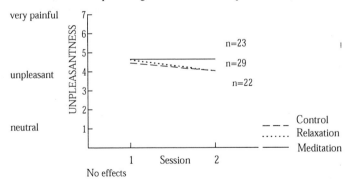

Both tables for Cardiac Subgroups show that the Accelerators had relatively higher ratings than their counterparts in both sessions.

Table 36.4 UNPLEASANTNESS of HI-Stimulus, C.Subgroup, Means & SE

Session	Accelerators		Non-Accelerators	
First	4.71	*0.28*	4.49	*0.24*
Second	4.52	*0.25*	4.02	*0.21*

3.6.2 State Anxiety (N=76)

The results for State Anxiety were similarly unexciting. There were no SM-Group factor differences ($F(2,70)=0.03$, $p=0.97$), and neither an effect for C.Subgroup ($F(1,70)=0.98$, $p=0.33$), nor for interaction of the two ($F(2,70)=0.63$, $p=0.54$). There was no Session effect at all ($F(1,70)=0.04$, $p=0.84$), no interaction with one of the between subject factors ($F(2,70)=0.05$, $p=0.95$ for Session X SM-Group and $F(1,70)=0.45$, $p=0.45$ for Session X C.Subgroup) and no 3-way interaction either ($F(2,70)=0.41$, $p=0.67$ for Session X C.Subgroup X SM-Group). The values for SM-Group and C.Subgroup can be read in Tables 36.5-6 below and the values for SM-Group are also presented in Figure 36.3. The Meditation Group had a relative increase of State Anxiety in the second session while both other Groups remained relatively unchanged.

Table 36.5 STATE ANXIETY, Stress Management Groups; Mean & SE

Pre Session	Meditation		Relaxation		Control	
First	39.76	2.24	40.53	2.01	39.62	2.25
Second	40.63	2.31	40.28	2.07	39.88	2.31

Figure 36.3
SM-Groups' Changes in State Anxiety before Physiological Experiment, N=76

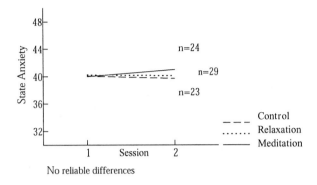

No reliable differences

The table for C.Subgroup shows relatively higher State Anxiety for the Accelerators.

Table 36.6   STATE ANXIETY, Cardiac Subgroups, Means & SE

Pre Session	Accelerators		Non-Accelerators	
First	40.79	1.80	39.57	1.62
Second	41.94	1.84	38.88	1.65

3.6.3 Mood after Stress Management Training

For the analysis the two between-subject factors C.Subgroup and SM-Group were employed. The within-subject factor was termed "Training" for changes following the instruction session in Stress Management. We looked first for Training effects and then for interaction effects of the between subject factors.

There were strong effects of Training on all three dimensions in the analysis with both between subject factors ($F(1,49)=92.17$, $p<0.001$ for *Distress*, $F(1,49)=45.39$, $p<0.001$ for *Appraisal* and $F(1,49)=7.22.$, $p<0.01$ for *Arousal*). There were neither interaction effects of the between subject factors in the overall means ($F(1,49)=2.24$, $p=0.14$ for *Distress*; $F(1,49)=1.85$, $p=0.18$ for *Appraisal*; $F(1,49)=0.47$, $p=0.50$ for *Arousal*) nor 3-way interactions with Training ($F(1,49)=0.01$, $p=0.94$ for *Distress*; $F(1,49)=1.71$, $p=0.20$ for *Appraisal*; $F(1,49)=1.14$, $p=0.29$ for *Arousal*). The are presented for single factor analysis.

Cardiac Subgroup

There was a C.Subgroup X Training effect for *Distress* ($F(1,51)=4.22$, $p<0.05$) but no main effect of C.Subgroup $F(1.51)=0.17$, $p=0.68$).The Training difference for the Accelerators was higher than for the non-Accelerators (Table 36.7).The initial difference between the Cardiac Subgroups was not reliable ($F(1,51)=1.78$, $p=0.19$, Figure 36.4). So, both methods had a stronger effect on the Accelerators' subjective level of *Distress* than on the non-Accelerators'.

Table 36. 7 DISTRESS **Cardiac Subgroups pre and post Training**

Cardiac Subgroup	$\overline{X}$ Pre	SE	$\overline{X}$ Post	SE
Accelerators	-0.48	0.70	-6.00	0.55
Non-Accelerators	-1.85	0.71	-5.15	0.56

Figure 36.4

Distress ratings before and after Stress Management for Cardiac Subgroups,

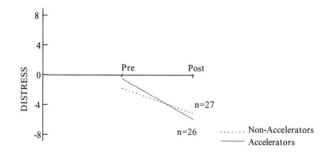

For *Appraisal* we had a reliable effect of Training X C.Subgroup (F(1,51)=4.04, p=0.05) with no main effect for C.Subgroup (F(1,51)=0.15, p=0.70). Again the Accelerators had started off with a "worse" mood (F(1,51)=1.01, p=0.32) but increased their *Appraisal* more than the non-Accelerators.

Figure 36.5

C.Subgroups' Appraisal ratings before and after Stress Management, N=53

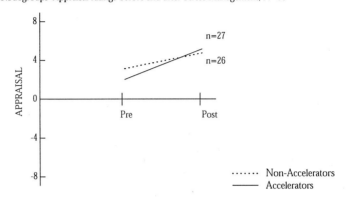

Table 36.8 for APPRAISAL, Cardiac Subgroup pre and post Stress Management

Cardiac Subgroup	$\overline{X}$ Pre	SE	$\overline{X}$ Post	SE
Accelerators	1.41	0.68	4.30	0.71
Non-Accelerators	2.54	0.70	4.12	0.73

There was no effect of C.Subgroup (F(1,51)=2.16, p=0.15) on *Arousal* but there were initial differences (F(1,51)=4.86, p=0.03) which were abolished after Training (F(1,51)=0.14, p= 0.72). The Accelerators felt more aroused before Training and reduced *Arousal* more than their counterparts. There was no effect for C.Subgroup X Training (F(1,51)=1.79, p=0.19) see Table 36.9 and Fig. 36.6.

Table 36.9 for AROUSAL, Cardiac Subgroup pre and post Stress Management

Cardiac Subgroup	$\bar{X}$ Pre	SE	$\bar{X}$ Post	SE
Accelerators	0.93	0.62	-1.37	0.76
Non-Accelerators	-1.04	0.65	-1.77	0.80

Figure 36.6

Cardiac Subgroups' Ratings for Arousal before and after Stress Management, N=53

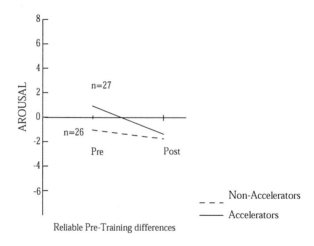

Stress Management Group

There were no interactions of Training X SM-Group on any dimension ($F_{(1,51)}=1.63$, p=0.21 for *Arousal*, $F_{(1.51)}=1.26$, p=0.27 for *Distress* and $F_{(1,51)}=0.94$, p=0.34 for *Appraisal*). There was an SM-Group effect for *Distress* on the overall mean ($F_{(1,51)}=7.77$, p<0.01) because the Relaxation Group was reliably less *Distress*ed overall than the Meditation Group. The pre-training difference was very significant ($F_{(1.51)}=7.17$, p=0.01). See the differences in Table 36.10 and Fig. 36.7.

Table 36.10 for DISTRESS, Ratings of SM-Group before and after Stress Management

SM-GROUP	$\overline{X}$ Pre	SE	$\overline{X}$ Post	SE
Meditation	-0.2	0.71	-4.80	0.56
-Relaxation	-2.36	0.66	-6.29	0.52

Figure 36.7

SM- Groups' Ratings of Distress before and after Stress Management, N=53

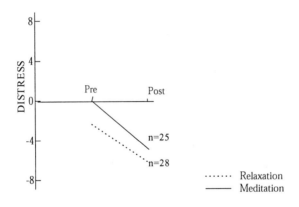

There was no overall mean SM-Group difference for *Arousal* (F(1,51)=2.00, p=0.16) and there was no SM-Group X Training effect (F(1,51)=1.63, p=0.21). The means suggested initial differences before Stress Management and that was confirmed by analysis (F(1,51)=4.44, p=0.04). The Meditators rated themselves *before* Meditation more aroused than the Relaxers did, but not so *after* meditation (F(1,51)=0.13, p=0.72 for post-Training mean difference). The meditation training had considerably reduced *Arousal* for some subjects but nor for all as the differences in values of dispersion show in Table 32.11. See also the graphic display in Figure 36.8.

Table 36.11 SM- Groups' Ratings of AROUSAL, before and after Stress Management

SM- Group	$\overline{X}$ Pre	SE	$\overline{X}$ Post	SE
Meditation	0.96	0.65	-1.36	0.79
PM-Relaxation	-0.93	0.62	-1.75	0.75

Figure 36.8

SM-Groups' rated Arousal before and after Stress Management

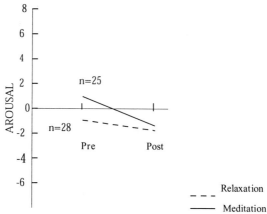

Reliable initial differences between Groups

Since these differences in ratings of subjective Arousal showed a tendency of Group differences it was looked for differences in the dimension's *items*. Differences at single-item-level would allow hypotheses on mood changing effects specific to the method. Analyses on all items were run and reliable differences were found for three.

There were in fact SM-Group X Training interaction effects for the *alert* (F(1,51)=5.88, p=0.02;Training: F(1,51) = 5.88, p=0.07; SM-Group: F(1,51)=0.64, p=0.43) and *sluggish* (F(1,51)=4.55, p=0.04; Training: F(1,51)=16.44, p<0.001; SM-Group: F(1,51)=0.76, p=0.39). The Meditators had increased considerably their alertness from 1.48 before to 2.00 after meditation while the Relaxers had slightly reduced from 1.93 (0.15) to 1.86

(0.16). *Sluggishness* in contrast decreased in both Groups but more in the Meditation Group namely by a difference of Δ=-1.08 from 1.76 (0.16) to 0.84 (0.18). The Relaxation Group changed by Δ=-0.29 only from 1.29 (0.15) to 1.00 (0.17). The initial differences were both significant at the 5% level.

For *Appraisal* we found a marginally significant overall mean SM-Group difference (F(1,51)=2.85, p<0.10). There had also been marginal initial SM-Group differences (F(1,51)=3.02, p<0.09) which did not change as dramatically (F(1,51)=0.98, p=0.33) as in *Arousal*. See Table 36.12 and the graphic display in Figure 36.9.

Table 36.12 SM Groups' Ratings of APPRAISAL, pre and post Training

SM-Group	$\overline{X}$ Pre	SE	$\overline{X}$ Post	SE
PM Relaxation	2.75	0.66	4.68	0.69
Meditation (n=25)	1.08	0.70	3.68	0.73

Figure 36.9

SM-Groups' Ratings of Appraisal before and after Stress Management, N=53

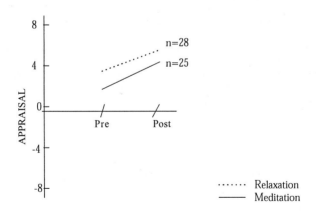

Multivariate Analysis of all Subjective Measures for C.Subgroup

The differences between Accelerators and non-Accelerators in the subjective measures pointed all into the same direction, namely towards lower tolerances on side of the Accelerators. They tended to have higher ratings in State Anxiety and Loudness and

Unpleasantness of HI-stimulus than the non-Accelerators. Furthermore, they tended to be more aroused, more distressed and had more negative appraisal than their counterparts before training in Stress Management. All those differences were not significant but it was possible that there was a significant common variance shared by all these variables. So, State Anxiety scores and ratings of HI-stimulus were taken from the first experimental session as well as the initial ratings on the mood dimensions. They were altogether analysed by multivariate analysis with C.Subgroup as between subject factor but there was no effect (Λ=0.91, F(6,52)=0.87, p=0.53).

Summary

Ratings of Hi-Stimulus did not reveal any significant differences. The Meditators had consistently higher ratings in the second session though than the other two Groups, particularly in Loudness of HI Stimulus.

State Anxiety did not show a trace of an effect either – again the Meditators had one point more on their scale before the second session

We had very significant effects of Stress Management training on all three mood dimensions but there were no SM-Group differences interacting with these effects There was, however, a tendency of the Meditators to tick more reduction of *Arousal* than the Relaxers. There were differences of SM-Group X Training at item level on this dimension for the items *alert* and *sluggish*. The Meditators had reliably greater changes after training than the Relaxers. The changes took different directions: the Meditators were more *alert* after training than before and the Relaxers less.

The C.Subgroup factor, in contrast, did interact with Training: We had two C.Subgroup X Training interactions, one for *distress* and one for *appraisal*. The Accelerators were less *Distress*ed after Training than the non-Accelerators. The same occurred for *Appraisal*: Initially lower *Appraisal* of the Accelerators changed into reliably higher *Appraisal* after Training. All Training effects were into direction of hypotheses - all subjects had gained lower levels of *Distress* and *Arousal* and more positive levels of *Appraisal*. Multivariate analysis of initial C.Subgroup differences in all subjective variables did not reveal reliable differences. The hypothesis had been suggested by directional unity of the values for Accelerators in these variables. Again the results were not left unaffected by a bias of non-random selection: the initial values for *Distress, Arousal* and *Appraisal* were reliably lower in the Meditation Group. That means the Meditators were reliably more distressed and aroused and had "appraised" also more negatively before training than the subjects of the Relaxation Group.

3.7 Personality / Temperament

3.7.1 Personality, Temperament and the Cardiac Defense Response (N=101)

Introductory Comment

Richard & Eves (1990) investigated whether physiologically based personality variables, i.e. variables independent of the stimuli eliciting the CDR, would predict individual differences in long latency. The scales of the Strelau Temperament Inventory (STI) and the Eysenck Personality Questionnaire were covaried with the subjects' heart rate of long latency post HI auditory stimulation and with their reflections in short latency. The idea of analysing covariance had been reversed by them: whilst covariance is usually analysed to partial out variance interfering with the investigation, Richard & Eves wanted to know whether there *was* covariance from an independent source other than the HI-stimulus variable. Analysis of covariance did then reveal negative correlations of heart-rate with Strength of Excitation (StE), Inhibition (StI), Mobility (M) and Extraversion (E) and a positive correlation with Neuroticism (N). Furthermore: significant covariance was also found for the differences of short latency. The correlations were measured at nominal scale level by t-test on Cardiac Subgroups' personality test scores and were then confirmed by parametric measurement. That is, heart rate response mean and trend-components (differentiating between Accelerators and non-Accelerators) of short and long latency post HI-stimulus were dependent variables and test scores were covariates. The pre-stimulus baselines were resting baselines and investigated as tonic measures separately. Scores on the lie-scale were also included in the investigation but only as a control variable for social desirability.

Since *phasic* heart rate responsivity here was at the focus within a similar paradigm as used by Richards & Eves, it is within the scope of this thesis to confirm their findings. By doing so it would have been more interesting to study personality covariance with *tonic* heart-rate changes of a longer sequence than they had used because this was now the main focus of stress related cardiac research (e.g. Obrist, 1982). The previous authors had analysed the peak- sequences of the two latencies, short latency over 5 sec and long-latency over 30 sec. Our analyses covered both peaks together and the deceleration between them (55 sec) as Eves & Gruzelier (1984) had demonstrated.

Therefore, the first attempt now was to confirm the results of the previous study at t-test level and in phasic heart-rate analysis of covariance. Then covariation with tonic responses having already been analysed for C.Subgroup differences earlier in this thesis were looked at. For phasic analysis the same sequence of short latency used by Richards & Eves was investigation, for tonic analysis, the entire HI-sequence covered by eleven 5-sec-windows plus baseline was the basis for covariance analysis with test scores. Both heart-rate sequences were run as dependent variables for the scores on each scale functioning as covariates by multivariate analysis of covariance. All analyses were run under one-tailed hypotheses. Lie scores were also included in the investigations but under the hypothesis that high social desirability responding, would be linked to lower heart-rate (see Introduction).

T-Test

A two-sample t-test was conducted with the two levels of the Cardiac Subgroups employed on all test scores. The values can be read from Table 37.1.

Table 37.1 T-test on Scores of Strelau's Temperament Inventory and Eysenck's Personality Inventory by Cardiac Subgroup

INVENTORY Scale	Accelerators (n=46)	Non-Accelerators (n=54)	T	p
STRELAU'S N=101 **Strength of**	Mean (SD)	Mean (SD)	Df 98	
-Excitation.	48.7 (12.3)	53.4 (12.5)	-1.89	0.03
-Inhibition	56.8 (12.2)	54.8 (10.5)	0.55	0.59
Mobility	53.2 (11.5)	58.3 (11.9)	-2.27	0.01
EYSENCK'S N=100	N=46	N=55	Df 99	
Neuroticism	13.8 (4.69)	14.4 (4.53)	-0.66	0.51
Extraversion	12.9 (4.18)	14.8 (3.55)	-2.51	0.01
Lie	1.2 (1.19)	1.09 (1.14)	0.45	0.65

The results confirmed the hypotheses on Strength of Excitation, Mobility and Extraversion. In contrast, Hypotheses for Strength of Inhibition, Neuroticism and Lie were not confirmed.

Heart Rate, Phasic and Tonic Response, and Personality

Individual HR-differences of first 5 seconds in short latency

Richards & Eves took the heart-beats from pre-stimulus baseline, and from 2nd- 6th second of response in short latency as dependent variables for their analysis. This sequence included the peak of the response of more than 83% of the subjects. In order to establish the differences in the trend-components of the polynomial contrasts we therefore had to run ANOVA on these five heart-rate values and pre-stimulus baseline respectively, with C.Subgroup as between and Time as within-subject factor.

Analysis showed C.Subgroup differences at mean level ($F(1,99)=14.32$, $p<0.001$) and over Time ($\Lambda=0.81$, $F(5,95)=0.001$). The Time differences were reflected in the linear

(F(1,99)=7.81, p=0.006), the quadratic (F(1,99)=14.83, p<0.001) and in the quartic trend-component (F(1,99)=3.70, p<0.03). The display of Figure 37.1 shows the heart rate from the 2nd to the 6th second post HI-stimulus by Cardiac Subgroups and their trend-differences. The trend differences explained together 24%, the response mean explained 12.6% of the models variance.

Figure 37.1 HR: Phasic Response sequence 5-seconds post HI-stimulus S1 at 60 sec post Warning; Acceleratory peak for 83% of subjects, C.Subgroup X Time Differences reflected in linear, quadratic and quartic trend-component; N=101.

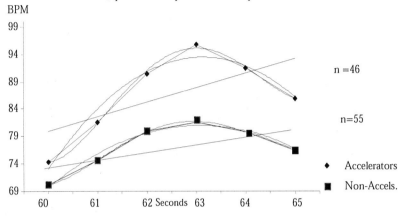

Personality and Phasic Heart Rate (Five seconds in short latency period)

Since the individual heart-rate differences of response mean and shape had been established, we were now able to test the hypotheses on covariance between test scores of STI and EPI scales. As in the previous study the pre-stimulus baseline and the heart-rate values of the first five seconds post HI-stimulus were transformed into the orthogonal trend components that had proven reliably different between Accelerators and non-Accelerators (linear, quadratic and quartic). The transformed heart-rate values were used as dependent variables, the test scores as covariates. The results are presented by row per test-score in Table 37.2.

There were reliable inverse relationships of the response mean with StE, StI and M and a positive relationship with N. So, high scorers on StE, StI and M had a lower cardiac response to the High Intensity Stimulus than low scorers on these scales. High scorers on N had a higher response mean than low scorers. In addition, the linear and quadratic trend-components were inversely correlated with the test scores. Low StE-, StI- and M-scorers had a more pronounced quadratic trend-component than high scorers, i.e they had a faster acceleration in their direct response to the HI-stimulus. There was a positive relationship for StE and M with the quartic component: High scorers had the faster directional changes in their sequences and thereby a more pronounced quartic trend component. There were similar differences for N: Heart-rate and test scores for N were positive linearly related and high N-scorers had a more emphasised quadratic trend, the indicator of faster heart-rate acceleration. The results for social desirability scores all went into the direction of hypothesis. There was an inverse relationship between socially desirable responses and acceleration of the heart-rate, however, the hypothesis was reliably confirmed in the linear trend-component only (r=-0.16).

Table 37.2 ANCOVA for Personality Test Scores with Heart-Rate of Phasic Response to auditory High Intensity Stimulus; N=101.

Covariate	Dependent Variables				
Scales	Response-Mean	Response-Shape described by Trend-Components			Multivariate Statistics
		Linear	Quadratic	Quartic	
STI	F(1,98), Pearson (r)				Λ, F(4,95),
StE	13.42** -0.35	3.67* -0.19	17.33** -0.39	3.13* 0.18	0.81, 5.58**
StI	10.43** -0.31	9.97** -0.30	9.95** -0.30	0.14 0.04	0.89, 3.08**
M	2.78* -0.17	0.49 -0.07	4.66* -0.21	4.98* 0.22	0.89, 2.95**
EPI	F(1,99)				Λ, F(4,96)
E	1.35 -0.12	0.23 -0.05	1.29 -0.12	0.52 0.07	0.98, 0.48,
N	7.80** 0.27	2.71* 0.16	7.56** 0.27	0.27 -0.05	0.92, 2.00*
Lie	0.39 -0.06	2.56* -0.16	0.77 -0.09	0.37 0.06	0.96, 0.99

(*)=P<0.06; *=P<0.05; **=P<0.01;

Personality and Tonic Heart Rate (Long Latency, 12 Five-Sec-Windows)

The same statistics as to phasic HR were now applied to response mean of tonic HR and the differentiating trend components Cardiac Subgroups. Resting baseline was analysed separately; see Table 37.3.

All results for the Strelau scales confirmed the hypotheses and the results from the phasic analyses: StE, StI and M again covaried inversely with the response-mean of tonic heart rate and additionally StI with the cubic trend-component. Hence, high scorers on StE and M had a lower cardiac response mean and high StI-scorers a lower response mean than low scorers and additionally a decelerative response shape.

Table 37.3 Tonic response heart-rate (5-sec-windows) to auditory HI-stimulus and Resting baseline in relation to personality test scores, ANCOVAs

Covariate		Dependent Variable				
Scales	Resting Baseline	Response-Mean	R-Shape (Trend-Component)		Multivar. Statistics
			Quadratic	Cubic	
STI - Strength of	F(1,98), r	F(1,98), r (Pearson)			Λ, F(3,96)
-Excitation	3.67*, -0.19	7.42**, 0.27	– 3.50 0.19	1.20 0.11	0.91, 3.30*
-Inhibition	9.97** -0.30	5.14** -0.23	0.00	4.57* -0.06	0.90, 3.38*
Mobility	0.49 -0.07	2.36(*) -0.15	1.99 0.14	4.28 0.21	0.93, 2.56*

N showed again a reliable but this time, confusingly, an inverse relationship with the response mean. Nevertheless, there was a positive reliable relationship with the quadratic trend-component (r=0.24). High N-scorers had the more powerful developed accelerative response shape.

Social desirability responses also shared variance with the shape of the Cardiac Defense Response: "Bad liars" also had a more developed quadratic component and "good liars" had less accelerative power in their response shape. However there was no evidence for the hypothesis in the variance of the response mean.

The resting baselines are also tonic measures and were therefore included into the table. They were reliably correlated with StE, StI, N and Lie but not with M and E.

Table 37.3 (cont) Tonic response heart-rate to auditory HI-stimulus and Resting baseline in relation to personality test scores, ANCOVAs

EPI	F (1,99)				Λ, F(3,97)
Extraversion	0.23	1.01	0.03	1.26	0.97, 0.91
	-0.05	0.13	-0.02	0.11	
Neuroticism	2.71*	2.96*	5.89**	1.14	0.92, 2.65*
	0.16	-0.17	0.24	0.11	
Lie	2.56*	0.20	3.52*	0.07	0.95, 1.58
	-0.16	-0.05	-0.19	-0.03	

(*) = P<0.06;   * = P<0.05;   ** = p<0.01

Summary

Correlation of physiologically based personality / temperament measures with cardiac defense was first tested on the basis of presence and absence of secondary acceleration. T-test confirmed that Accelerators had reliably lower scores on the scales for Strength of Excitation, Mobility and Extraversion. There was no confirmation for the hypotheses on Neuroticism and Strength of Inhibition with this method.

The test scores also covaried directly with heart-rate of phasic and tonic measurement, although not consistently with T-test results, and not with all three aspects of heart-rate either (response mean, response shape and resting baseline).

Covariance with the phasic response mean confirmed T-test for StE (-0.35) and Mobility (-0.17) with reliable correlations but not for Extraversion (-0.12). On the other hand the response mean of short latency did confirm the predictions for Strength of Inhibition (-0.31) and Neuroticism (0.16).

So, low scorers on Strength of Excitation, Strength of Inhibition and Mobility (regarded as "weak" individuals by the approach of the Russian School) had significantly higher response means in their phasic response to High Intensity auditory stimulation than high scorers ("strong" individuals). These results found also support from covariations of test scores with the response shape. Strength of Excitation, Strength of Inhibition, Mobility and Neuroticism covaried with the quadratic component; i.e. low scorers on the Strelau scales had a more pronounced quadratic trend-component in their HR-sequence and therefore a response shape reflecting faster acceleration. Conversely high scorers on Neuroticism had a more pronounced quadratic component. Furthermore, all already mentioned scales except Mobility but including Lie covaried with the linear trend. There was a lack of reliable covariation with the quartic trend-component reflecting decelerative responses (because of faster approaching directional turning points). Such positive covariation was produced by analysis for StE and M only. High scorers had a more pronounced quartic trend-component.

Covariance with the response mean of tonic heart-rate from the 55 seconds post stimulus sequence was consistently related to the Strelau scales, although Mobility only marginally. Neuroticism was also inversely related and therefore against the direction of the hypothesis. On the other hand, Neuroticism had a reliable relationship with the resting baseline and the quadratic trend-component. The response shape did not play a role for the Strelau scales but the resting baseline as tonic measure was correlated with Strength of Excitation and Strength of Inhibition. Social desirability scores were also positively related to baseline and quadratic component: High social desirability scorers had a lower resting baseline and less acceleration of the heart rate than low scorers.

3.7.2 Personality and Choice of Stress Management

The research task involving the STI and EPI was orthogonal to the task on Stress Management. Nevertheless, since we had investigated systematically the differences between subjects allocated to the three Stress Management Groups, it was tempting to add psychometric features to the psychophysiological profiles. Hypotheses had been developed from the research body that prospective Meditators were more neurotic and more introvert than prospective non-Meditators (see Introduction 1.6.3).

Firstly we wanted to investigate whether there was a relationship between the test scores and the allocation to the Groups by using One-way ANOVA for the test score variables with the three levelled factor SM-Group (Table 37.4-5).

Table 37.4	Scores of prospective Stress Management Groups on Scales of Strelau Temperament Inventory, Means, SD		
SM-Group	St of Excitation	St of Inhibition	Mobility
Meditation	48.1 2.1 *	54.4 2.1	52.7 2.0 (*)
Relaxation	50.4 1.9	55.0 1.9	57.3 1.9
Control	56.6 2.4	59.5 2.3	59.5 2.3

(*) marginally significant, * significant at p<0.05

Regarding the Strelau scales the SM-Group factor had a reliable effect only on StE (F(2,97)=3.70, p<0.03) and a marginally reliable effect on Mobility (F(2,97)=2.65, p<0.08). The Meditators scored lower on both scales than the Control Group (Tukey's pairwise comparison: p=0.02 for StE; p<0.08 for M).

Regarding the Eysenck scales, differences were found for social desirability (F(2,98)=5.68, p<0.01): Tukey's pairwise comparison of probabilities showed very significant differences between Meditators and the two other Groups who responded obviously more in a consensus oriented style (p=0.01 for both comparisons). There were no other effects or near effects in the test score variables of the EPI. Thus the hypotheses on Anxiety/Neuroticism and Introversion were not confirmed.

One observation was made consistently across both scales: obviously the extreme values were taken by Meditation and Control Group while the Relaxation Group took consistently the middle position. However, the scores of the Relaxation Group were predominantly closer to the scores of their Stress Management competitors than to the no-SM-Controls. Only for Neuroticism the mean distances were about the same, in Mobility the Relaxation Group scored near the Controls as on all other scales (Excitation, Inhibition, Extraversion and lie) they scored at a similar level as the Meditators. So it appeared we had a continuum of nervous system properties on which each Group had its own range and the ranges of the two positive Stress Management Groups were positioned more closely together. The continuum included the lie scale and by adding a glance at the dispersion values, the Relaxation Group was more homogenous than the Meditators but both were outscored by the Controls showing the highest dispersion.

Table 37.5	Scores of prospective Stress-Management Groups on Scales of Eysenck's Personality Inventory, Means, SD		
SM-Group	Extraversion	Neuroticism	Lie
Meditation	13.6 0.7	14.4 0.8	0.91 0.19 * *
Relaxation	13.9 0.6	14.7 0.7	0.93 0.17
Control	14.4 0.8	13.0 0.9	1.77 0.22

** significant at p=0.01

This is all worth to be noted because psychometric similarity and difference of the Stress Management Groups mattered in the context with the further above investigated physiological differences in the averaged sequences of warning biased by non-random allocation to Stress Management.

As we know from the previous section higher phasic heart-rate responsivity to HI-stimulation covaried reliably with StE test scores. It therefore was not useful to test covariation of StE scores with minor SM-Group differences on phasic heart-rate as we had tested StE covariation with C.Subgroup differences. The C.Subgroups had already explained the major part of the variance, hence the covariance with low SM-Group differences would have been only trivial in this context.

Summary

Prospective Meditators were not reliably more neurotic than prospective non-Meditators as it had been suggested by the literature. However, prospective Meditators scored significantly lower than Controls on the scale for Strength of Excitation and marginally lower than Relaxers. In Pavlovian terms they had a weaker nervous system than Controls meaning their nerve cells could sustain less stimulation.

It was observed that in all but one scale, namely Neuroticism, Meditators and Controls took the extreme positions and the Relaxers' Group means were closer to the Meditators than to the Controls except for Mobility. Dispersion was highest for Controls and lowest for the Relaxers, suggesting selection bias in the active stress management group.

3.7.3 "Dropping Out" (Attrition)

Dropping out and the Cardiac Defense Response

Of the 101 subjects who performed the first experimental session 78 completed the second session after 4-6 weeks of Meditation, PMR or no-Stress Management. This represents a dropout-rate of 22.8%. The proportions were 13 Accelerators, 9 Equivocals and only one Decelerator. No significant differences were found for the two-levelled category used throughout the study (Chi^2 (1)=1.45, Fisher's test: p=0.24; Table 37.6).

Table 37.6	Frequencies for Cardiac Subgroup (row %) by Dropouts and Continuers					
Cardiac Subgroup	**Dropouts**		**Continuers**		**Total**	
Accelerators	13	28.3%	33	71.7%	46	100%
Non-Accelerators	10	18.2%	45	81.8%	55	100%
Total	23	22.8%	78	77.2%	101	100%

From the Stress Management Groups there were 11 PMR, 10 Meditation, and only two Control subjects on the drop-out list. For further analysis the Control subjects were removed from the sample because they had had no involvement with Stress Management. An interesting question was how the Cardiac Subgroups were distributed over the two stress-management Groups (the two Control Dropouts were from both categories). The cells were pretty evenle distributed as can be seen in Table 37.7.

Table 37.7	Frequencies for C.Subgroup by Dropouts in SM- Group, % for Table			
Cardiac Subgroup	**Drop-Meditation**		**Drop-Relaxation**	
Accelerators	6	28.6%	6	28.6%
Non-Accelerators	4	19.0%	5	23.8%

Physiological differences had not been investigated up to date but questionnaire data had revealed psychosomatic differences between Meditation Dropouts and Continuers (Smith, 1983). The Accelerators had been represented by a third more among the Dropouts than among the Continuers although this was not enough to produce a significant difference at nominal scale level. Hence it was not unlikely that we would find differences in heart-rate by using the more powerful instrument of analysis of variance. Therefore, the Continuers were matched with the Dropouts according to Cardiac Subgroup and age and, with one exception, by gender (there was one more male subject in the Continuers /Meditation sample because there was no female subject's record left in the sample). Hence we had a sample of 42 subjects, (2x10 for Meditation and 2x11 for PMR Continuers and Dropouts respectively).

Tonic Heart-Rate differences (5-sec-windows) of the first session's stimulus periods (Warning and High Intensity) were calculated by ANOVA with the between subject factor ConDrop (Continuers/Dropouts), SM-Group (Relaxation/Meditation) and Repetition (2) and Time (12) as within subject factors. There was a reliable difference of ConDrop in the overall mean $F(1,38)=4.55$, $p=0.04$; ($\overline{X}_{DROPOUT}$ =78.4bpm, $\overline{X}_{CONTINUE}$ =71.1bpm). There was no effect for SM-Group ($F(1,41)=1.61$, $p=0.21$) and no interaction of the between subject factors ($F(1,38)=0.38$, $p=0.54$). At within-subject level we had a Repetition effect ($F(1,40)=4.88$, $p=0.03$), a Repetition X Time effect($\Lambda=0.53$, $F(11,28)=2.32$, $p=0.04$) and an all-factor interaction of Repetition X Time X ConDrop X SM-Group ($\Lambda=0.54$, $F(11,28)=2.29$, $p=0.04$). The Factor-Time-differences were mirrored in the quadratic trend-component ($F(1,38)=4.01$, $p=0.05$) suggesting differences between Dropouts and Continuers in one of the Groups. The first sequence was then tested for the Meditation Group but confirmed only marginal effects for ConDrop in the response mean ($F(1,18)=3.79$, $p<0.07$) and the quadratic trend-component ($F(1,18)=3.52$, $p<0.08$).

Figure 37. 2 HR: Tonic Response of Continuers and Dropouts in prosp. Meditation Group to first HI-Stimulus - Marginal Effects in R-Mean and Quadratic Trend

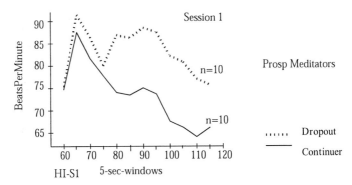

However, the all-factor interaction effect was not confirmed by post-hoc test of hypothesis (ConDrop X Time) in either of the SM-Groups ($\Lambda=0.33$, $F(11,8)=1.46$, $p=0.30$ for Meditators; $\Lambda=0.45$, $F(11,10)=1.09$, $p=0.45$ for Relaxers).

The response mean differences between Continuers and Dropouts of the Meditation Group in the graphic of Figure 33.3 seemed predominantly linked to the Cardiac Subgroup differences in the long latency period. Since differences of long latency had been reflected in short latency the phasic response post first HI-stimulus was also analysed with the same factor design for effects on the eleven second-by-second HR-values.

Phasic heart-rate differences were not found for the ConDrop factor, neither in the response mean ($F(1,38)= 2.57$, $p=0.12$ for between subject effect) nor for the measure-points over Time ($\Lambda=0.72$, ($F(10,29)=1.16$, $p=0.36$ for ConDrop X Time). There were no reliable differences either between the Dropouts within Meditation or Relaxation Group of short latency ($F(1,38)=0.07$, $p=0.80$ for ConDrop X SM-Group, $\Lambda=0.72$, $F(10,29)=1.14$, $p=0.37$ for ConDrop X SM-Group X Time).

Warning sequences, tonic response: The factors had no reliable between subject effects on the time-variables of warning ($F(1,38)=2.18$, $p=0.15$ for ConDrop; $F(1,38)=0.75$, $p=0.39$ for SM-Group and $F(1,38)=0.41$, $p=0.51$ for Interaction). There were no interactions with the within-subject factors either ($F(1,38)=2.04$, $p=0.16$ for Repetition X SM-Group X ConDrop; $\Lambda=0.85$, $F(11,28)=0.47$, $p=0.91$ for Repetition X Time X SM-Group X ConDrop; Time effect: $\Lambda=0.44$, $F(11,28)=3.25$, $p<0.01$). Hence we found no differences in anticipatory responses to an impending HI-stimulus . See Table 37.8.

Table 37.8 for ANOVA on physiologically based Personality Measures for Dropouts and Continuers and Stress Management Groups

Scales	CONDROP $F(1,38)=$	SM-Group		ConDrop X SM-Group
STE	1.19, p=0.28	0.13	0.722	2.55, p=0.12 r=-0.25
StI	1.46, p=0.24	0.00	0.974	0.02, p=0.88
M	0.01, p=0.94	0.97	0.331	0.30, p=0.59
EXTRA	0.72, p=0.40	0.03	0.861	1.30, p=0.26
NEUR	2.63, p=0.05 r=-0.25	0.05	0.821	0.82, p=0.37
LIE	0.00, p=0.99	0.00	0.99	0.11, p=0.75

Dropping out and Personality / Temperament

For psychometric differences between Dropouts and Continuers overall and in SM-Groups Anova was run on all psychometric variables with the factors ConDrop and SM-Group. There were no significant effects for all but one of the models: N was tested under one-tailed hypothesis and post-hoc test confirmed higher scores for subjects who dropped out of the experiment than for those who continued ($F(1,40)=2.96$, $p< 0.05$; $\overline{X}_{DROP}=15.95$, $\overline{X}_{CONT}=13.76$,). Dropouts in the Meditation Group tended to score lower on StE than Continuers ($r=0.25$ for both). See Table 37.9 and Figure 37.3.

Table 37.9	Personality Scores for Dropouts and Continuers, Means and Standard Error					
	STE	StI	M	NEUR	EXTRA	LIE
Continuers	49.86	57.67	54.57	13.76	13.29	0.95
N=21	2.56	2.60	2.29	0.90	0.99	0.23
Dropouts	45.52	53.05	55.05	15.95	14.38	0.94
N=21	2.56	2.60	2.29	0.90	0.99	0.23

Figure 37.3

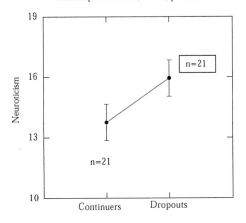

Scores on Neuroticism (EPI) by Continuers and Dropouts
Least Squares Means, N=42, p=0.04

Summary

Physiologically Dropouts had a higher overall mean heart rate than Continuers in their tonic response to HI-stimulus with repetition. They had marginally higher scores on Neuroticism tested under one-tailed hypothesis ($r=0.25$). Such psychophysiological parallelism could not be found for the differences within the Meditation Group: here Dropouts had a marginally higher overall mean and a more pronounced quadratic trend than Continuers (under two-tailed hypothesis) but psychometric differences were found only within the Relaxation Group: Dropouts here had marginally lower scores on Strength of Excitation ($r=0.25$) compared to the Continuers.

4. Discussion

4.1 Individual Differences in Heart Rate Changes and Concomitant Variables, Hypothesis 1

Proportions of Individual Differences here and in other Studies

The non-parametric categorisation procedure resulted in 32 Accelerators (41.6%), 8 Decelerators (10.4%) and 37 Equivocals (48%). If we consider the small differences of stimulus strength and the subjects' age range, then the proportion of Accelerators emerging from this study is very consistent with the proportions found in the previous studies with normal subjects. Richards & Eves (1991) found 33.3% Accelerators with 110dB tone and Eves & Steptoe (1986) found 39.2% with 105dB white noise. Eves & Gruzelier (1984) found a higher ratio of 50% Accelerators with 127dB tone (equal to our white noise 110dB, Graham, 1975) with a sample of 14 undergraduates with an age range from 18-21 years. There is, however, a marked difference in the proportion of Decelerators found in the different studies. Eves & Gruzelier (1984) found 36%, Eves & Steptoe (1986) 19.6% and Richards & Eves (1991) had 11.6% which comes closest to our figure. The decline seems to be a negative function of the year the studies were run. (The experiments for this study were run from the beginning of 1990 to summer 1991).

Sequences of High Intensity Stimulation

We found our hypotheses on individual differences between subjects in response to high intensity stimulation confirmed by ANOVA. Individual differences of the Cardiac Defense Response were found for the sample of 101 subjects in the first period of long and short latency and in the five seconds post stimulus in short latency containing the *accelerative peak* of 83% of the subjects[13]. The differences were found in the univariate statistics for the response mean, in the multivariate statistics for the time-variables and in the models testing polynomial contrasts for the response shape. Analysis of tonic response for the two-session-complete-sample also confirmed the hypothesis.

Interestingly there was a reliable C.Subgroup difference in the Repetition sequence (C.Subgroup X Repetition X Time effect) of the respiration rate data: The Accelerators had taken one respiratory cycle less than the non-Accelerators. This could be a sign of reduced metabolism in the repetition period at the time when the secondary acceleration was habituating. Furthermore, the Accelerators had consistently a lower respiration-rate except in the repetition warning sequence where both cardiac subgroups were equal. Both phenomena suggest cardio-somatic de-coupling and therefore the individual differences were rather directly centrally triggered than indirectly by respiratory influences.

The individual heart rate differences of the long latency period and direct response to the HI-Stimulus found no confirmatory effect in the time-variables of blood pressure. It should be mentioned, however, that Systolic Blood Pressure was consistently but not significantly higher (by 0.4, 0.9. 1.7mmHg) for the Accelerators throughout the first session's three

---

13 This result has been reported at the beginning of the Personality section.

values. In Diastolic Blood Pressure the picture was consistently reverse: The Accelerators had lower values (by -1.9, -0.8, -.9 mmHg) than their counterparts. This is consistent with the findings that people respond either with their heart-rate or with their vascular system, also known under the dichotomy of vascular and cardiac reactors (Turner, 1994).

Neither the time variables of EMG nor SCL reflected cardiac subgroup differences in the first session. Concerning EMG this is in contrast to the reference study of Eves & Steptoe (1986/7) and could have to do with different analyses. They had analysed the response in "one go" while this analysis was done separately for startle, phasic and tonic changes. There were no comparison data for SCL.

The Russian School had delivered evidence for „weak" individuals having lower sensory thresholds than „strong" ones (with regard to the capacity of their nerve cells to sustain stimulation) and therefore higher intensity stimuli will have a stronger impact on the nervous system (for reference see Richards & Eves, 1991). The latter argued that the subjective ratings in their results (and also of Eves and Gruzelier, 1984) contradicted this threshold hypothesis.

There were also no reliable differences in our subjective ratings of the HI-stimulus characteristics and in the scores of Spielberger's state anxiety test, taken before the physiological experimental sessions. The ratings for all cognitive variables (loudness and unpleasantness of HI-stimulus, State Anxiety and Mood) showed that Accelerators were more sensitive to stimulus characteristics, scored higher on state-anxiety and had "worse" mood values than non-Accelerators consistent with direction of hypothesis. However, there were no reliable differences found in multivariate analyses. All these results together confirm the results of previous research on normal participants (Eves & Gruzelier, 1984; Richards & Eves, 1991).

Sequences post Warning of an impending High Intensity stimulus

There was no convincing evidence for reflection of individual differences in both sequences of anticipation of an impending High Intensity-stimulus as the above authors had reported. Some evidence for sensitisation could be inferred from cardiac subgroup differences found in the averaged means of the warning sequences. That is because these differences reflected a widening gap of the cardiac subgroups in the repetition period. When the C.Subgroups' sequential HRs are being compared in Figures 31.8a,b, relative differences can be observed within the range of 71 to 75 bpm in the first warning sequence (a) increasing in the repetition sequence (b). In the work of Eves & Gruzelier (1984) the non-Accelerators showed a pronounced deceleration of the heart rate in response to the first Warning. Our data, in contrast, did not suggest any differences of that kind.

Cardiac Subgroup differences were also found in the warning periods of SCL and EMG but they were not parallel effects to HR: The EMG showed session differences in the overall mean of startle to Warning because the Accelerators had sensitised to warning in the second session. A similar but more conspicuous effect appeared in the variables of SCL: The direct response in SCL to the first presentation of Warning stimulus in the second session showed reliable differences over Time (Session X Repetition X Time effect) with differences in the linear and cubic trend. The Accelerators had raised their levels faster and higher than the non-Accelerators. All these physiological results from the sequences post warning showed a tendency of the Accelerators of sensitising towards anticipatory stimulation. There will be more comment on the possible role of the SCL result at the end of this section. Before that the major role the warning sequences played in this study has to be discussed.

Firstly: Analysis had shown lack of evidence for presence of cardiac subgroup differences in the first warning sequence and sensitisation of those in the repetition sequence. From that „mishap" of our data followed that the hypothesis on specific effects of stress management on Accelerators in the warning sequences of the second session (see section Hypotheses) could not be tested in the comparison of sessions. Secondly: The warning sequences (of the impending aversive white noise high intensity Stimulus) are of psychological relevance because assumed psychological impact of the warning stimulus (of an impending aversive stimulus) is measured by the physiological response and that means it will be likely to reflect anticipation fear with little contamination of cardio-somatic coupling. The latter, in contrast, would be more the case in an active avoidance task and indeed in the High Intensity sequences where also the sensory impact of the physical stimulus is reflected, particularly in the short latency period. Thirdly: The warning sequences bear also more relevance for the paradigm than those of HI-stimulus. That is because the earlier found reflections of the long latency cardiac subgroup differences in them would link the paradigm to the construct of cardiac reactivity and make the paradigm therefore useful for further research on cardiac reactivity as a *temporally stable* construct (Turner, 1994)[14].

So, the non-replication of cardiac subgroup differences in anticipation of an impending HI-stimulus is disappointing in every possible respect. Finally: the Cardiac Subgroup differences in anticipation of the highly aversive stressor have not been replicated by any other experimenter than by Eves in his studies for a Ph.D. However, it perhaps has not been tried either by anybody else than by the author of this thesis for a Ph.D. Since in this study the differences related to the periods of high intensity stimulation could be replicated in detail (long latency, short latency and first accelerative peak), why not this one?

One could argue that in a clear passive coping paradigm this effect was only documented once (Eves & Gruzelier, 1984) and only with twelve subjects. In our reference study, which has not been published in detail (e.g. Eves & Steptoe, 1987) the subjects engaged in video-games while they were expecting the high intensity stimulus. It was neither a purely classical conditioning task (as such a passive task) nor was it an active-avoidance task but it was something between the two. Since our physiologically based temperament questionnaire data confirmed evidence for non-Accelerators being equipped with a „stronger" nervous system, it is likely that they were distracting themselves with ease by playing video games. Quite in contrast the "weaker" and therefore more anxious Accelerators were less able to do so and so the difference in anticipation fear was able to show. In our purely classical conditioning passive paradigm the lack of distracting games may have made the non-Accelerators focus on their inner signals of fear (Pennebaker, 1982). This may have been the case particularly in combination with another inter study difference explained in the next paragraph.

There was a difference between the reference studies and this one in the instruction style of the experimenters: The experimenter of this study did not want to have the subjects in

---

[14] inter-task consistency and laboratory-field generalization

doubt about the *very* disturbing character of the noise because that she would have regarded as unethical. At the time the author of this thesis started her experiments passionate discussions of ethical issues like instructing subjects clearly were going on in the department (spring term 1990). Therefore she felt strongly obliged to emphasise the slightly nasty character of the HI-intensity stimulus thereby scaring the non-Accelerators. A detached style of instruction certainly would have been more in line with the other studies than her perhaps overly sympathetic instruction style.

4.2 CDR and Dis-habituation, Hypothesis 2

There is one hypothesis left about the cardiac subgroup factor: Dis-habituation of differences in the first HI-sequence after an inter-session-interval of 4-5 weeks. We would have expected differences to re-appear in the control group because they had no stress management during the interval. However, there was no sign of C.Subgroup differences in any of the Groups since we had no effect for the 5-way interaction (Session X Repetition X Time X C.Subgroup X SM-Group).

4.3 Individual Differences of the CDR and Personality, Hypothesis 3

Summary

Correlation of physiologically based personality / temperament measures with cardiac defense was first tested with the criterion of presence / absence of secondary acceleration. T-test confirmed that Accelerators had reliably lower scores on the scales for *Strength of Excitation, Mobility,* and *Extraversion.* Hence Accelerators were more introvert than their counterparts, they were less able to do long lasting and intensive work and had less capability to recover after fatigue and intensive activity. Finally they showed less persistence and ease of coping with obstacles (*Strength of Excitation*), had less capacity to switch from one activity to another and were more inhibited in social contacts (*Mobility*). There was no confirmation for the hypotheses on *Neuroticism* and *Strength of Inhibition* at this level of analysis.

Covariance with the *phasic response mean* confirmed the T-test for *Strength of Excitation* (-0.35) and *Mobility* (-0.17) with reliable correlations but not for *Extraversion* (-0.12). Also in line with the T-test was the negative result for social desirability. On the other hand, the response mean of short latency did confirm the predictions for *Strength of Inhibition* (-0.31) and *Neuroticism* (0.16) but was inconsistent with the T-test result. The discrepancies between the different measures will be explained later in context with other inter-study differences.

The hypotheses on covariation of test-scores with the *response shape* were also confirmed by this study: *Strength of Excitation, Strength of Inhibition, Mobility,* and *Neuroticism* all covaried with the quadratic component. Namely, low scorers on the Strelau scales had a more pronounced quadratic trend-component in their HR-sequence and therefore a response shape reflecting faster heart-rate-acceleration suggesting a more „efficient" defense system in terms of activation. Conversely, high scorers on *Neuroticism* had a more pronounced quadratic component. Furthermore, all already mentioned scales except *Mobility* but including *lie* covaried with the linear trend. On the other hand, there was a lack of reliable covariation with the quartic trend-component for *Neuroticism* and *Strength of Inhibition* suggesting that only accelerative behaviour of heart rate be reliably related to these test scores. Such positive covariation was produced by analysis for *Strength of Excitation* and *Mobility* only. High scorers had a more pronounced quartic trend-component.

Covariance with the *response mean of tonic heart-rate* from the 55 seconds post stimulus sequence was consistently related to the Strelau scales, *Mobility* only marginally though. Neuroticism was also correlated, but inversely, and therefore against the direction of the hypothesis. On the other hand, *Neuroticism* had a reliable positive relationship with the resting baseline ($r=0.27$) and the quadratic trend-component ($r=0.16$).

The response shape of tonic response did not correlate with the Strelau scales but the resting baseline, a tonic measure, was correlated with *Strength of Excitation* and *Strength of Inhibition*. Social desirability scores were also positively related to baseline, the linear component of phasic response and the quadratic component of tonic response: High social desirability scorers had a lower resting baseline and less acceleration of phasic and tonic response than low scorers.

Commonalities and Differences of the two Studies

Since our results have to be discussed in context with the study of Richards & Eves a table will be useful to show the commonalities and differences at a glance. Columns represent the studies, rows the aspects of heart rate.

Table 4.0: Inter-study comparison [1] of significant correlations between aspects of the Cardiac Defense Response and physiologically based personality scales

	Correlations for test-scores significant at 5% level			
Aspects of CDR	**RICHARDS & EVES 1991** **Lie tested in T-test only**		**Jung-Stalmann**	
C.Subgroups (T-test)	StE, StI, M, E, N, -		StE, -[2], M, E, -,	
Baseline (Resting)	StE, StI, -, E, N		StE, StI, -, -, N, Lie	
Response-Aspect	Phasic	Tonic	Phasic	Tonic
Response -Mean	StE, StI, M E, N	StE, StI, - E, N	StE, StI, M N, -, -	StE, StI, (M) -, -, -
Trend-Component 1,2,3,4 (linear– quartic)	-, -, -, -, -, -,	StE2, -, M2[3] -, -	StE1,2,3 StI1,2, M2,3 N1,2, -, Lie1	-, StI3, -, -, N2, Lie2

[1] Effects are indicated in the cells by the scales (abbreviated) and their order
[2] Sign (-) for missing effect in place of scale
[3] Effect into opposite direction of hypothesis: high scorers had more pronounced quadratic trend

Most striking are the commonalities found for *Strength of Excitation, Strength of Inhibition,* and *Neuroticism*: both Strelau scales covaried with heart-rate directly, namely with the response means of both latencies and with the initial resting baseline.

The most striking differences are found in the cells of phasic response trend-components with missing effects overall in the older study and the most „hits" in this study. More important though are the differences for *Neuroticism* (tonic mean and T-test) and *Strength of Inhibition* (T-test). These scales were not significant in the just described cells of this study and *Extraversion and Mobility* did not have correlations with any of the response means, which was implied already in the description of the commonalities. *Neuroticism* covaried in both studies with the phasic response mean and with the resting baseline. All personality/ temperament scales were correlated with the C.Subgroup categories in T-test of the older study while in our study only *Strength of Excitation, Mobility* and *Extraversion* can be found in that cell. Hence, *Strength of Excitation* had the most and *Mobility* and *Extraversion* the least commonality in the comparison.

Finally, there was no confirmation for *Extraversion* directly covarying with heart-rate at all.

Differences in Results follow from Inter-Study Differences

Before we discuss further the confirmatory results - mainly those on *Strength of Excitation* and *Strength of Inhibition* - we want to consider the differences in *Neuroticism* and *Strength of Inhibition* in T-test and tonic response mean and then the differences in *Mobility* and *Extraversion* in the response means. The former inconsistency of the two studies can be explained for both latency periods by taking into account the inter-study differences

➢ of structure and strength of the stimulus,

➢ of the data sampling of the tonic data, and finally

➢ of the number of subjects.

Our study used a double-stimulus of 110dB white noise and that is equivalent to 128dB tone (see section on OR, DR and startle, Introduction). In the older study only a single 110 dB tone was employed and that was only equivalent to 100 dB white noise. As Eves & Gruzelier (1984) have demonstrated, the number of Accelerators increases linearly with stimulus strength up to 122dB tone with no further increase at 127dB. Thus we would have expected a lower percentage of Accelerators in our study. In fact Richards & Eves (1991) found 33.3% Accelerators by using 110dB tone and we found 41.6%. From Eves & Gruzelier (1984) follows that the scores of those 8.3% more Accelerators in our study realised their „accelerative potential" under the more extreme stimulus conditions of 110 dB white noise respectively 128 dB tone and would not have been calculated in this category under 110dB tone conditions. Therefore we want to call these 8.3% in our context „high-threshold-Accelerators".

Furthermore and following the hypothesis that low *Strength of Inhibition* and high *Neuroticism* goes with secondary acceleration and that there is some linearity in the covariation of test scores with responsivity, the high-threshold-Accelerators scored higher on *Strength of Inhibition* and lower on *Neuroticism* than the majority of Accelerators („low-threshold-Accelerators"). To put it more simple: Even people with higher levels of *Strength of Inhibition* and lower levels of *Neuroticism* will respond with a secondary acceleration of their heart-rate when the stressor almost hits the pain threshold. That means a third of the Accelerators' test scores of this study would have been in the non-Accelerator category of the other study, thus explaining the lack of effect in T-test for *Strength of Inhibition* and *Neuroticism*. The relative mean differences were even into the other direction of hypothesis.

Secondly, by the same token it is reasonable to assume that the high-threshold Accelerators were at the „bottom" of a secondary acceleration and therefore their lower HR-values would reduce the response mean of secondary Accelerators. This and the perhaps relatively insensitive 5-sec-window sampling method used for the tonic sequence may have affected the negative outcome at mean level, and even a reliable difference into the opposite direction of hypothesis. This tendency showed already in the T-test result based on tonic heart-rate differences in the long latency period.

Also, by the same token, the relatively high scores on *Strength of Inhibition* and low scores on *Neuroticism* of the high-threshold-Accelerators did not affect the covariation with the mean of the short latency period for two reasons: The measurement was at full interval scale level (compared to T-test), and we had second-by-second sampling of heart-rate as in the reference study. Finally, there were 25% more subjects in this study than in the other. All three factors provided more variance and could counterbalance the relatively lower heart-rate of the high-threshold Accelerators.

Let's finally look at the noticeable differences in trend-component analysis. We said above that our high threshold Accelerators had pulled down the response mean of their own cardiac subgroup because they lowered the bottom of secondary acceleration. But still they had a secondary acceleration like the others, namely significantly more heart-beats in the category 4bpm above baseline (see Methods). That is confirmed by the very reliable correlation of *Neuroticism* scores with the quadratic trend-component of tonic response (Table 37.3).

So, what about the results in *Strength of Excitation* being affected by the just described threshold differences for secondary acceleration? In fact the results give support to our theory: the high-threshold Accelerators were supposed to have higher scores on that scale than the majority of low threshold Accelerators. We had a discrepancy of response mean and quadratic trend in tonic response: Whilst the scores covaried inversely with the response mean, they did so positively with the quadratic trend-component. At first sight this is puzzling but not in the light of our interpretation: 8 or 10 of high StE scorers had a secondary acceleration under the conditions of ultimate stimulus strength. However, it was a lower one than the majority had and therefore it did not affect the differences of the response mean.

In the same context we can see the inter-study differences in *Extraversion*. We had a positive result at T-test level but no correlation with heart-rate changes directly, noteven with the response mean. Since *Extraversion* is correlated with *Strength of Excitation* we have to explain that difference in order to be consistent with our assumption, and that should not be a problem considering differences between the *Extraversion*-scales of the

EPI and the EPQ. The latter does not include a scale measuring impulsivity, which became part of the scale measuring psychoticism, the third dimension of Eysenck's personality theory (e.g. Eysenck, 1987). It is likely that the difference was due to this lack of variance in the *Extraversion*-scale of the EPI. Furthermore, the discrepancy between the studies is also consistent with Stellmack & Gelhorn (1991) who claimed that differences in *Extraversion/* introversion show usually in response with milder stressors.

The extreme stimulus-strength used in our study also explains the involvement of more correlation with trend-components. We had in both phasic and tonic responses more correlations. The greater difference in the cell of phasic responses has also been contributed by the difference in subject numbers: 25% more in this study.

Finally the difference in the response key of the questionnaire, dichotomic forced choice in the ear*lie*r study, and a three-options-key (yes / no / don't know) in this study, must have had an effect too. For example those with high *Strength of Inhibition* may have more often chosen the "don't know" option than low scorers and so may have subjects high on *Neuroticism*.

For the hypotheses on social desirability scores we did not find clear and unequivocal evidence for related lower cardiac responsivity. If we had we would have found effects involving the cardiac subgroup factor. Nevertheless, we found resting baseline and trend-components of lower phasic and tonic cardiac responsivity of self selected groups was reliably linked to higher *lie* scores. Hence there is not a both-way but a three-way relationship of compliance with social consensus (working for exams), *lie* scores and cardiac responsivity. That indeed is in line with the studies of Kiecolt-Glaser & Greenberg (1983), Brody, Veit & Rau (1997) and Kline et al (1993), described in Introduction. The former studies had used mental arithmetic tasks testing links between *lie*-scores and cardiac responsivity with different outcomes. Kiecolt-Glaser *et al.* admitted their MA-task through the experimenter and thus the positive result had a bias of social interaction. Brody *et al* used a computer-advised task and had a negative outcome. Kline et al conducted a physiological experiment on high and low *lie*-scorers and found smaller auditory evoked potentials in the EEG-response to high intensity stimulation (104dB tone).

However, it is not surprising that people who comply more with social consensus thereby avoiding external psychological stressors are quieter in their cardiac responsivity. Perhaps that is related to results on social support reducing cardiac responsivity in stress tasks (see Turner, 1994) with implications for social learning during infancy.

The CDR, the STI and an Intriguing Field Study

This study adds to the evidence about the reflections of the CDR in Personality traits of physiologically based constructs describing behaviour patterns that are stable over time. This hypothesis had been successfully put to the test by Richards & Eves (1991) and their conclusions can stand for these results too, namely

> "…Individuals who exhibit marked defensive responding are likely to be easily disrupted by a variety of intensive and/or stressful conditions (*Strength of Excitation*) and may have little capacity for quick reaction, diversity and flexibility" (p. 1005).

Richards & Eves (1991) in the Discussion of their results replicated here, raised the hypothesis about adaptiveness of the Defense Response. Their and our results seem to prove that <u>not</u> those individuals who are well-prepared and well-organised for stressful events and show behavioural restraint display the CDR more often. On the contrary those who are easily disrupted by such events do display the CDR as the covariation of low *Strength of Excitation* scores with higher responsiveness to intensive stimulation suggests.

That is in line with a double-blind field study on performance under highly stressful conditions made by the Teplov- Nebylitsyn school in the sixties (Gurevich, 1966) reported by Strelau (1983, p.53). The study looked at the interrelations between strength of the nervous system and work performance of the operators in a simulated breakdown in a power plant. Results suggested

„the behaviour of all persons with a weak NS [nervous system] to be disorganised during the breakdown emergency. This was reflected in numerous aspects of behaviour, and especially in disorders of perception, memory, and thinking. Subjects with a strong NS... displayed considerable endurance in the face of stress. The differences between these two groups were found to be significant" (Strelau, p.53).

While the strength of the NS was assessed on the basis of a seldom-used physical stimulus (critical frequency of flashing phosphene), work-performance was measured behaviourally by experimenters who were not aware of the physiological results. There are other studies quoted by Strelau reporting similar correlations between strength of the nervous system and real life situations, (e.g. professional activity and school performance). One laboratory study simulating high environmental stressor levels remains to be reported in this context.

In an experiment on sensory deprivation Strelau, Sosnowski *et al.* (1986) put young soldiers individually for six hours into a dark room, restrained them with belts to a chair and measured heart rate and skin resistance (SR) at 14 time points. There were reliable differences between high and low *Strength of Excitation* scorers in SR at 13 time points, but not in HR. A second, threatening condition was created in a low-pressure chamber simulating a peak comparable to 5000 metres altitude. Low scorers had lower SR values than high scorers. Also in this condition HR of low and high scorers showed no reliable differences. The heart seems indeed only to separate the populations when the challenge is sudden and an extreme threat as in the simulated conditions in the field study.

As in all the previous studies we had no reliable differences of subjective stress level. In our study the noise ratings of the Accelerators were relatively higher both for loudness and unpleasantness but the differences did not even remotely approach significance. However, there is physiological evidence that „weak" individuals have lower sensory thresholds than „strong" individuals and therefore stimuli of the same intensity have a stronger impact on weak individuals (Gray, 1964). Hence in our data we would just have found the same contradiction of physiological and subjective data from the same subjects as it is common in psychophysiological research.

Support for Eysenck's Hypothesis

High scorers on Neuroticism showed reliably more cardiac responsivity to high intensity auditory stimulation. They had higher tonic heart-rate (baseline), more phasic responsivity (short latency mean and shape), and more cardiac acceleration in tonic response. The lack of tonic response mean differences in our study has been explained by a floor effect of secondary acceleration following elicitation through most extreme stressor-intensity. That line of explanation was consistent also with differences <u>and</u> commonalities in other scales, e.g. Strength of Inhibition. Our results on Neuroticism by and large therefore replicated Richards & Eves' findings and therefore added evidence to Eysenck's hypothesis that under extraordinary stressfull circumstances individual differences in Neuroticism will affect physiological activation as far as heart-rate is concerned.

Fahrenberg's null hypothesis is now difficult to be upheld: The negative results in multivariate studies were based on the use of comparatively mild, active coping stressors as mental arithmetic task and cold pressor test. Walsh, Wilding & M. Eysenck (1993) even found less increase in HR with more neurotic subjects also in a mental arithmetic task.

At questionnaire level differences in emotionality or Neuroticism have always been obvious in the literature and therefore Eysenck's breakdown hypothesis of the „arousal-activation barrier" always remained in the foreground of the interest into stress research. Because of the negative evidence for physiological correlates Fahrenberg (1992) considered the possibility that Neuroticism was purely a subjective trait. In the same context he questioned the testability of the Eysenck hypothesis on ethical grounds. Therefore the individuals who participated in our studies cannot be appreciated highly enough for their contribution to knowledge gained in this field of individual differences. This background adds further importance to our results replicating earlier found correlations between Neuroticism scores and the cardiac Defense response.

Somewhat puzzling is the correlation with resting baseline heart-rate in both studies. It actually questions the tonic character of that baseline and suggests it being an early anticipatory response to the impending threat.

Social Desirability, Cardiac Responsivity and Self-Selection

Lie scores were directly correlated with cardiac responsivity: The resting baseline was inversely correlated (r=-0.16) and so was the linear trend-component of phasic response in short latency and the quadratic trend-component (r=-0.19 for both) of tonic response involving long latency. So, high *lie*-scorers had a lower resting baseline and a less accelerative shape in their phasic and even more in their tonic response than low scorers. This result confirms previous results on this issue of high lie scorers lowered responsivity: Brody, Veit *et al.* (1997) found an inverse relationship of lie scores and cardiovascular responsivity to stressful (mental arithmetic,) and pain dampening (baroreceptor, for HR-deceleration) stimulation. High lie-scorers showed lower cardiovascular responsivity to computer-advised mental arithmetic (with SBP) and baroreceptor stimulation (with HR). Decelerative responsivity to pain dampening stimulation is a predictor for self-measured development of hypertension over 19 months (see references in Brody,Veit *et al.*, 1997) and interpreted as support for the operant development of hypertension.

Our result is closely connected to the findings of Kline et al (1993) who tested the hypothesis that high defensive individuals as indicated by the EPQ (lie scores ≥ 7) diminish the impact of high intensity stimuli at the level of the cortex. The investigation was based on the assumption that „defensiveness represents a predilection for the attenuation of stimuli that are too intense for an individual" (p. 8). Their study demonstrated that high lie scores were associated with reliably smaller auditory evoked potentials[15] by high intensity auditory stimulation (94dB and 104dB tone) in comparison to low scorers (lie<7). High defensive subjects showed significantly lower amplitudes to high intensity tones (94, 104dB Tone) at sites of the frontal lobe and the vertex than low scorers. The frontal lobe is associated with affect and consciousness and that made their results in context with defensiveness and repression particularly interesting. The authors suggested this process being a strategy of desensitisation used by defensive individuals. Here lies one important difference to our paradigm: The tones of four different intensities were repeatedly presented at random and the subjects could not anticipate when the painful intensities were due to occur. Therefore the process of diminishing stimulus-impact was suggested to occur non-consciously.

There is also a difference between the subject-samples of the two studies: None of our subjects was defensive the maximum value was 5 and so within the criterion of low defensiveness in the comparison study. Our lie-scores were even extremely low ($\overline{X}$=1.14, SD=1.16) which can be explained by the fact that most of the participants were psychology students and on their guard towards this well known test. Therefore perhaps also the effects were not more impressive and did not cover a wider range of aspects, i.e. differences between Accelerators and non-Accelerators in T-test. Furthermore, we used a noticeably higher intensity and that could have made less high scorers respond low (than with a lower intensity) and thereby may have also worked against the hypothesis. Therefore our results are even more confirmatory for the EEG results. The relationship between lie scores and cardiac responsivity seems to be robust also at the lower end of the scale and the upper end of responsivity.

After having dealt with the psychological and physiological aspects of social desirability scores our second result links lie scores indirectly to cardiac responsivity and encompasses the behavioural aspect. The no stress management control group had lower heart-rate levels over time in the averaged means of the warning sequences than relaxation and meditation group. The differences were significant in comparison with the meditators. Secondly: The control subjects had reliably ($p<0.01$) higher *lie* scores than both meditators and relaxers. It is not difficult to find a behavioural parallel to social desirability scoring in the control subjects' profile: control subjects wanted to comply with two social expectations confronting them: achieving good results in their exams by focussing on their academic work and showing a collaborative attitude to the research needs of the psychology department without having to bother with daily training sessions in stress management. Looking at the psychological-behavioural profile and their reliably lower expectancy heart-rate (and relatively lower heart rate overall) in comparison with the meditators one could come to the strictly behavioural conclusion that compliance with social expectation is a good prevention of cardiac hyperactivity.

---

[15] transient electrical activation of cerebral cortex regions associated with audition

Relevance to Clinical or Health Psychological Issues

This study was based on the assumption that if cardiac reactivity is a predictor for hypertension personality/temperament measures could be used for identification of high-risk future hypertensives. That hypothesis was developed predominantly from animal research in the beginning of the eighties (Folkow, 1982). However, Turner (1994) cautiously stated in reviewing the literature, "no definitive evidence links cardiovascular reactivity with hypertension [in humans]" but that "several lines of evidence, when considered together, suggest inferentially that associations may exist between reactivity and hypertension, and which therefore encourage continued research." (Turner, 1994, p60). However, a later 4-year longitudinal study (Brody, Veit & Rau, 1996) found no evidence for the reactivity hypothesis. In a sample of 75 normotensive German subjects who had performed a 90-sec serial subtraction task with an interpersonal stressor component, no correlation was found with mean blood pressure taken after 4 years. Surprisingly *Neuroticism* was inversely linked to the development of hypertension, i.e. the more emotionally unstable one is, the less one is prone to develop essential hypertension. The author quoted supportive evidence from other studies, which linked experimental suppression of sad feelings with increased sympathetic activation of the cardiovascular system and low blood pressure with "neurotic" complaints. If we consider the negative result on cardiac reactivity together with the inverse relationship of *Neuroticism* with longitudinal elevated mean blood pressure, then the data of the two studies showing *Neuroticism* as positively linked to the CDR, fit in neatly with the re-discovered old hypothesis that "emotional suppression results in psychosomatic disorder" (Alexander & French, 1946, cit Brody, Veit *et al*, 1996, p 378). This makes *Neuroticism* viewed as "generalized emotional reactivity within limits … desirable from the cardiovascular psychosomatic perspective" (Brody, Veit et al., ibid.). Conversely we can state that the results of Richards & Eves (1991) and of this thesis would contradict Brody *et al.*'s results about the negative relationship of *Neuroticism* with hypertension if the reactivity hypothesis with respect to development of hypertension were true.

4.4 Effects of Stress Management Factor Hypotheses 4,5

The chronology of the hypotheses mirrors the process of research. However, for the discussion it is necessary to change the order because a selection bias has to be considered before factor effects are discussed. Therefore hypothesis 5 is treated before hypothesis 4.

4.4.1 Profiles of Prospective Stress Management Groups and Dropouts, Hypothesis 5

Since the methodological rule of random allocation to the stress management groups could not be kept we had the disadvantage of having to control a possible selection bias. This was not too difficult because the design included two measurements, one before and one after training in stress management (which has not been done in the few comparable studies). Additionally we had the advantage of being able to generate physiological and psychometrical profiles of the prospective members of groups from the data of the first session. While there is ample documentation of questionnaire data on anxiety and *Neuroticism*, „there has been a paucity of research on personality variables in relation to the practice of meditation" as Delmonte (1987b) wrote in his review. No physiological profiles of prospective meditators have been found in the research literature. Therefore first the physiological profiles are discussed and then concordance (and discordance) are searched for in the psychometric data.

Physiological profiles

Prospective stress management groups: higher tonic anticipatory response levels

The prospective meditators' averaged HR means of the anticipation periods were reliably higher than those of the controls at mean level as well as over time (expressed in cubic and quadratic trend differences, see Figure 31.1a). The ranking order of response level of this sequence represents the relative inter-group differences in HR of the first session with the meditators on top, the controls at the bottom and the relaxation group in the middle position. There had been no reliable group differences in respiration rate or EMG and that allows us to exclude somatic coupling. Hence, it is suggested that the prospective meditators exerted more sympathetic influence in their response than the subjects of the control group did and hence psychological processes were involved.

There was a similar result in the SCL- data for both meditators and relaxers: In fact, there was a reliable difference in baseline shift from resting to recovery baseline between both stress management groups and controls: Prospective meditators and relaxers had an increase in recovery baseline. Hence, they were more sympathetically activated in expectancy of the second warning stimulus than the controls were. This was also reflected in elevated HR levels in the second warning period, which contributed, together with initial differences, to the group differences in the averaged means of both periods. So, those who were more interested in learning stress management techniques had more sympathetic activation than those who were less interested in relaxation or meditation! The psychological profiles will show that they also had higher subjective stress levels.

Control group had higher diastolic blood pressure and skin conductance levels

There was also a paradox in the SCL-data that has to be considered: The prospective control group started with slightly higher resting baselines and higher SC- levels than the other groups during the warning periods (again aggregated means). It could be argued that since the control group was at relatively higher resting baseline levels the law of initial value could have moderated the differences in recovery baselines. However, between subject differences in SCL recovery-baseline were normal and the events in the HR warning periods supported the higher responsivity of prospective stress management groups compared with no-controls.

We did not use continuous monitoring of blood pressure changes and so our BP time variables (taken at entering the laboratory, pre, and post physiological experiment) were by no means parallel to the other physiological data. The changes in SBP from initial baseline to resting baseline could be a contribution to measuring expectancy, and, similarly, from resting baseline to post experiment value recovery. However, apart from relative differences in the initial baseline (the controls being higher than the meditators and relaxers) there were no differences in the first session. But reliable differences were found in the diastolic values: the no-stress management control group had higher diastolic values throughout the first session and their Accelerators had an atypical positive shift from initial to resting compared to their equivalents in the stress management groups. This led to further differences of the pre and post experiment mean and overall. The higher diastolic values of the control subjects indicated their vascular system having more tonus in the relaxed state of the cardiac cycle than the other groups. It is suggested that this finding be in line with the slightly higher SC-levels. The controls were perhaps in a more alert state because they were more ambitious and focussed on their work tasks than the stress management groups and therefore had higher tonic levels of DBP and SCL.

Psychological profiles

In fact, the meditators turned out to have a "weaker" nervous system than the control Subjects by scoring reliably lower on the *Strength of Excitation* scale and marginally significant lower on the *Mobility* scale. So, this is in line with their higher initial HR, particularly in the averaged means of the warning periods. There were no reliable differences at all for *Extraversion*. TM-meditators have often been found being reliably more introvert than non-meditators (e.g. West, 1980; Delmonte, 1987b). Here the difference in the techniques (listening and chanting plus mental vs purely mental) may have had an effect. It makes sense that more introvert people are drawn to a very quiet technique and a more active and even noisy technique will repel those more introvert individuals. Moreover, the meditators were asked to participate in weekly group meditation and that might have attracted more gregarious individuals who are by definition not introverted.

Another difference from reference research (Williams, Francis *et al*. 1976, West 1980) was found for *Neuroticism* and Spielberger's state anxiety. There were no appreciable differences at all and this also contradicts the above physiological differences in the warning periods. This could be explained by the dual component theory of anxiety (Schalling *et al*, 1995) which Schwartz, Davidson & Goleman (1978) used as basis for their dual process theory of relaxation and which has been found valid for research on meditation (Delmonte, 1987). Thus the anxiety of the meditators was more somatic and less cognitive. Schalling's studies also showed that *Extraversion* correlated only negatively with cognitive, and not with somatic anxiety, which is in line with our results. Schwartz *et al.* claimed evidence for their dual process theory by physical exercisers showing reduction of somatic anxiety and TM-meditators having cognitive anxiety reduced. These results were flawed because no random selection had been practised. But taken all together (TM-meditators being more introvert, ASDY meditators not but more somatically anxious) their study may have proved that somatic anxious people chose somatic stress management techniques and cognitive anxious people chose cognitive techniques. However, to date there seems nothing like an identity of psychometrical and physiologically assessed anxiety phenomenon. Strelau (1992) stated „that when psychometric and physiological data are compared, not only are different measures of anxiety used but also different kinds of anxieties are being compared" (p. 2).

We found participants from the self-selected control group scoring significantly higher on the lie scale than both meditators and relaxers. This finding has been discussed in context with lower physiological responsivity of this group in the first section on personality variables.

Psychophysiology of dropping out

Subjects who discontinued the investigation by not participating in the second physiological experiment are named here as dropout subjects or short as dropouts as it has been done in another publication quoted by Delmonte (1980).

The data were searched for psychometric and physiological differences between continuers and dropouts of both stress management groups. First of all the dropout rate was low (22.7%) compared to other studies involving meditation; West referred to 50% and sometimes 90% (West, 1987). As to the psychometric differences, the TM-related results of the previous two decades on meditation-dropouts could not be confirmed perhaps because of the small sample-sizes that were used for the comparisons (n=10) where the scores tended towards the direction of the hypothesis. The overall difference for dropouts and continuers was marginally reliable for *Neuroticism* only. Thus the tendency of being trait-anxious for individuals dropping out of meditation practice within a short trial meditation has been confirmed but not for being more introvert or state anxious, than continuers. The scales of the Strelau Temperament Inventory were tested for the first time and the differences were not significant for *Strength of Excitation* and *Strength of Inhibition* but pointed into direction of hypotheses though.

The physiological differences were slightly more impressive. There was a quadratic trend difference superimposed over marginally reliable overall mean differences between continuers and dropouts of the prospective meditation group (with two-tailed hypothesis). There had been an overshoot of 1.5 Accelerators in the dropout sample of the meditation group and this contributed largely to those directional differences in the long latency period (Figure 37.3), but that cannot have been the only contributing factor. These results at least support the hypothesis that dropouts from a larger sample of self-selected meditation subjects have a heightened responsivity to novel high intensity stimuli. There is a parallel to be drawn to a correlation of cognitive sensitisation and short term dropping out of meditation practice. Delmonte (1988) investigated a clinically anxious outpatient sample treated with non-cultic TM over a period of two years. Those patients who had scored high on a repression - sensitisation scale (more specific information not given by the author) were reliably more likely to drop out after all time points of compliance measurement (2,3,6,12,24 months). Similarly, *Extraversion* was negatively correlated with attrition. At all measurements the dropouts were reliably more introverted than the continuers.

It cannot be suggested that our dropouts were from the same population as the TM-dropouts. The appeal of a chanting meditation technique must be different from that of a purely mental technique (which is probably why we had those difficulties with random allocation to the meditation group). This difference also explains why we did not find the meditators more introverted than the PMR subjects.

The discrepancy of psychometric and physiological emotionality between the groups is interesting. While the relaxation-dropouts were reliably higher on *Neuroticism* than their continuing colleagues, we had these phasic HR- differences between dropouts and continuers in the meditation group. As already mentioned, the continuers of this group had shown a higher overall responsivity during the warning sequences of the first session suggesting that physiologically emotional individuals were predominantly attracted to this ASDY-meditation technique. However, the most responsive individuals dropped out suggesting avoidance of the high intensity stimulation lying ahead in the second experimental session.

4.4.2 Effects of Stress Management Training, Hypothesis 4

No basis had been found in the data for testing the main hypothesis - stress management training effects on Cardiac Subgroup -, we identified instead physiological selection effects on the variables for the first time as discussed in the previous section.

The meditation group's two major patterns of heart rate changes after 4-5 weeks of stress-management training have to be explained, ideally along with two single effects regarding respiration-rate and skin conductance levels. These effects were:

➢ Baseline shift and anticipatory activation

➢ Fast Habituation of recovery baseline with Session and Repetition

➢ Habituation in phasic heart rate

➢ Respiratory effect in parallel

➢ SCL increase of Meditators/Accelerators

➢ No recovery SM-Group differences by minimum heart rate comparison

➢ Cognitive differences between Relaxers and Meditators after one session of stress management.

The list of effects above suggested no session effects of the training in progressive muscle relaxation. Trends and indirect evidence for impact of PMR will be discussed prior to the effects of meditation training.

Some evidence for activation reducing effects by Progressive Muscle Relaxation

There was some evidence for activation-attenuating affects within the PMR-group in the heart rate resting baselines, in systolic blood pressure.

The relaxers had a clear heart rate habituation effect in the second session to repetition of HI-stimulus compared to the control subjects (p=0.04) and unlike the meditators they had not increased their initial resting baseline. They also had reduced their post experimental SBP by 4.1mmHg while the meditators had increased theirs by 1.25mmHg and this together led to Session differences between the two groups. There had been, however, no reliable differences between them and the control group who had also slightly reduced SBP but only by 0.4 mmHg. These effects of training in progressive muscle relaxation are the only ones found and should not be underrated considering the lack of control over training and the baseline differences with the control group. The hypothesis, however, on cardiac responsivity reducing effects of PMR in a period over 4-5 weeks regarding heart rate other than baseline has to be rejected. Of course, the question for possible reasons arises and answers can be found.

In the forerunner study of this investigation (Eves & Steptoe, 1987/86) the reduction of HR-acceleration occurred only in the physiologically more responsive Accelerators (through a 48 hours inter-session interval with 2-3 training sessions in PMR). In our sample almost half the number of subjects (43%) were categorised as higher responsive ones, but the extension of the treatment time did not result in a similar effect as described by the authors of the previous study.

On the basis of the reviewed studies Borkovec & Sides (1979) suggested to take subjects from clinical populations whose high activation levels are a contributing factor to their illness. The problem of this study was that the prerequisite hypothesis of the design was not confirmed: that Accelerators would show reliably higher physiological activation in the anticipation period of high intensity stimulation. The short-term effects of brief PMR-training found by Eves & Steptoe had been based on those anticipatory physiological differences found in their sample.

The negative outcome might also be connected with lesser motivation to practice the exercises regularly over a time period of 4-5 weeks, at least once a day. It could be argued that taped instruction has proven as not successful as Borkovec & Sides suggested. In fact, the instruction had been given only in one individual therapist guided session whereas the daily practising followed taped instructions. This was also the procedure in the Eves & Steptoe reference study. However, practising along with a tape over four weeks requires a higher level of persistent motivation than practising twice within 48 hours. Therefore it is concluded that weekly single sessions would have had to be included in order to achieve better compliance. Unfortunately, such a measure would have required more resources than were available to the author of this thesis.

It is known from other studies that meditation appeals more to the subjects´ readiness to practice than relaxation does (Lehrer *et al*, 1983). Another aspect may also have fostered the higher level of motivation for the meditators: The weekly group meetings to introduce the meditation technique to the new subjects also had a socialising character. The experimenter tried to organise group meetings as check- ups for the relaxers in order to produce equality of condition in this respect. Those meetings were not attended by more than two at a time and often not attended at all. That may well have to do with the „*alerting*"character the meditation technique had which distinguished the effects the two SM techniques had from each other. Consistent with that PMR made the relaxers feel more *sluggish* as will be discussed later in more detail.

Having said that this study cannot contribute much evidence to cardiac activation reducing effects of PMR applied over a month's time, it should be noted that we found indirect evidence for effects that PMR (and ASDY meditation) had on the subjects' organisms. In the warning sequences of repetition, we found session changes of within-group variability in measure heart rate and that in it suggested effects stress management had had on the subjects. The active stress management groups had clearly reduced their variability and the no-stress management control group had not (Fig. 31.12a,b). These changes seemed to have „blocked" a Session X Repetition X Time X SM-Group effect (see end of session comparison, Fig. 31.11-12). The marginally reliable effects between all groups over time (p=0.07) in the repetition sequence of the second session suggested attenuation of anticipatory activation for the relaxation group. The time differences between controls and relaxers were reflected by differences in the quartic trend-component because of a distinctive decelerative phase in the response of the relaxation group (Fig. 31.11a, 232.5 sec - 247.5 sec). In that phase, their heart-rate variability was at its lowest level (Fig. 31.12b). The meditation group, in contrast, had at the same time a predominantly accelerative response also simultaneous with a within group variability-low. Beforehand we need to see our results in the light of other studies recently published.

By reviewing the studies of the previous decade under the key words PMR and heart rate, only one study out of five confirmed the hypothesis of cardiovascular reactivity reducing effects of PMR. All of these studies were conducted on clinical populations, mostly hypertensives, and did not involve stress experiments except one: Amigo, Gonzalez *et al.* (1997) investigated 45 patients with mild essential hypertension in a longitudinal study over eight weeks under three conditions: PMR, isotonic physical exercise, and a placebo control group. Cardiovascular responsivity was assessed in a mental arithmetic task and an exercise task. PMR was superior to exercise and placebo in heart rate at a six months follow up assessment only, but not yet after eight weeks!

Another study with patients in phase II cardiac rehabilitation (Collins & Rice, 1997) did find after 6 weeks of training significant differences in resting heart rate and systolic blood pressure between experimental and control group. The relaxers had reliable within-subject reductions in mean resting heart rate being also 8.6 bpm reliably lower than that of the controls. However, the Control Group showed the lower systolic and diastolic blood pressure values.

It is suggested that short-term effects after a few times of practice of progressive muscle relaxation, as shown in the Eves & Steptoe study, but perhaps of any stress management method, may always carry some placebo effect in their variance.

The rest of the discussion will be dedicated to the results of meditation training, starting with the single features of the technique and relating them to literature in the past. Then the more recent research on controlled breathing will be applied and consistencies between those and our results will be shown starting with the remarkable result in respiration rate.

Heightened Expectancy Fear of Meditation Trainees

Let's come to the heart of the matter.

The meditation group had a shift in resting-baseline, a tonic measure, of 5.7 bpm heart-rate in the second session followed by time effects in the tonic and phasic values. There was a hidden session effect in the tonic averaged warning sequences: differences over time between meditators and relaxers in the second session. This difference was not expressed in the main analysis because it was „camouflaged" by first-session-differences between meditators and controls and all those differences added up to a SM-Group X Time effect in the main analysis. The controls namely had increased their response in the second session while the relaxers had slightly attenuated their response. The meditators however responded from a higher plateau because their resting-baseline was elevated after 4-5 weeks of training. This baseline shift and its consequences gave rise to the hypothesis that meditation rather raises anticipatory physiological fear of an impending high intensity stressor than lowering it. The phasic response showed more conspicuously the effects of that baseline shift, again in its averaged means, with a Session X Time X SM-Group effect (Fig. 31.10b) showing differences between Meditation and Control Group. Meditation affected Accelerators' phasic SCL

In the second session the cardiac Accelerators had sensitised in their skin conductance levels within 15 sec post (averaged) warning. Interestingly, they had had the lowest initial levels of all groups in the first session and developed their 'responsivity potential' only after meditation training. That showed in a C.Subgroup X SM-Group X Session X Time effect of the first three 5-sec-windows and contributed secondly to the C.Subgroup differences overall of this sequence (Fig. 35.6/7). The Control group's Accelerators had also slightly increased their electrodermal responsivity in the second session and that had contributed to the effect too. The relaxation-Accelerators, in contrast, had relatively reduced their responsivity as already mentioned above.

Thus the results from SCL suggest that the ASDY- meditation technique increased anticipation arousal of the Accelerators who, however, had had the lowest initial SCL-values in the first session compared to the other cardiac subgroups. Since the non-Accelerators did not further increase their initial higher levels (on the contrary, see Fig. 35.7) it seems that the meditation technique had had a balancing effect here towards a more alert state in the sequence of anticipation (which then continued throughout the other stimulation sequences). On the other hand, PMR had a relatively reducing effect on Accelerators' SCL, while practising-no-technique at all in the control condition obviously increased further the SCL of the already in the first session more responsive Accelerators. These findings seem complementary to the results on anticipation in the main variable heart-rate.

Effect common to different techniques: Habituation instead of Sensitisation

What would David Holmes in Kansas have said about this increase in activation? It would probably be „raised anxiety levels" that he had alluded to in reviewing (1984/87) the Goleman & Schwartz study (1976). Even without his obvious bias against oriental meditation techniques he would probably dismiss meditation as a useful stress management technique. An elevated baseline, he might say, is not a good thing at all and he may have a point there given that lowering levels of activation generally seems the solution to stress. Also in Yoga teachings it is regarded as a sure sign of spiritual progress if a student can do without excitations of the autonomous nervous system and a beginner will not be expected to show such signs of progression on his path to enlightenment.

Let us resort to Lazarus & Averill's (1972) claim as Goleman & Schwartz did before us: Raised physiological values in expectation of a fearsome stimulus are only then causing problems to health if they sensitise (see section on Holmes in Introduction). Our meditators' recovery baseline after first HI-stimulus impact had habituated markedly by 3.8 bpm and significantly ($p<0.001$) more than the baseline of the control group who had raised their recovery baseline by 1.2 bpm. The difference between this second session's recovery and the resting baseline of the first session was negligible (-1.8 bpm) and therefore the data gave us a clear indication for the meditators' healthy response to High Intensity stimulation (as they did for the relaxation group, $p=0.04$). Furthermore we had another recovery effect rather than sensitisation in the phasic responses to HI-Stimulus. There was a Session X Repetition X SM-Group effect in the phasic means showing an impressive change in the response to repetition (Fig 31.9). Of course we have to consider that the phasic response contains startle in the first three seconds, habituating by definition.

Let us summarise. Elevated baseline and response-mean of the meditation group's first warning and high intensity sequences suggested higher somatic expectancy fear towards the first high intensity stimulus of the second session. However, normal habituation of recovery baseline after warning repetition was consistent with Goleman & Schwartz' interpretation of faster recovery of a threatening stimulus linked to heightened physiological activity in anticipation of that stimulus. The former was preparing for action in anticipation of the threatening stimulus, the latter the appropriate response to the absence of a real threat.

It is therefore suggested that in a passive coping situation diverse meditation techniques as the passive TM-technique as well as the active multimodal ASDY-meditation technique, enhance a preparation-for-coping-response in anticipation of a threatening stimulus. Such diverse meditation techniques also enable the meditators to adjust their anticipatory activation quickly to an appropriate level. In the next paragraphs it will be shown that results in other physiological and psychological variables also support a healthy character of the meditators' heart-rate changes in response to the stressors of the second session applied after training in ASDY-meditation technique.

Differences between the studies explaining recovery differences

Goleman & Schwartz had found faster recovery from the impact of the accident-film-stressor in terms of minimum heart rate after stressor impact but we did not. We found only habituation of anticipatory activation after identifying an effect as regression to the mean. On the other hand both studies were about anticipating a stressful stimulus, why the difference in recovery?

First of all: the high intensity stressor with passive coping used in our study was harder to cope with than an accident-film. Our design aimed at getting distinguishable individual differences in cardiac responses, which in high responders elicited a secondary acceleration even between 15 to 55 seconds post stimulus impact. Passive anticipation of a highly aversive noise is more than waiting for a horrific sequence in a film. The occupation with watching the sequences before can be regarded as a sort of active coping.

Then: Both our studies used self-selected meditators but the TM-*siddhas* (as long-term practitioners are called in TM-jargon) had an experience of two years and that means that further selection had taken place. The high cardiac responders may have dropped out, a hypothesis that would be supported by our physiological data on attrition: meditation-dropouts had a higher response-mean and a more pronounced quadratic trend-component shown their response-shape of the first HI-sequence (p<0.08, see Figure 37.2). There may well be a trait effect as well. The *siddhas* had perhaps learnt to recover quickly as our short-term meditators had within normal habituation limits (compared to the first session).

Finally, Goleman & Schwartz (and likewise Lehrer et al.'s studies) used only a one-session-design in order to avoid habituation effects to the stressor. In our case one could argue that the meditators had 4-5 weeks time to build up some anticipatory fear with their practice of visualisation and listening to the sound within. It would also make sense that PMR rather diminished the anticipation fear by practising progressive muscle relaxation for the second test.

Lehrer *et al.* (1983) hinted at the possibility of the *cognitive focus* of meditation being the cause for the meditators' raised *cognitive* anxiety expressed by higher ratings of the most fearsome moment during the stress experiment with a 100dB tone as stimulus (*p.661*). Our meditators, in contrast, had *physiological* anxiety in anticipation of the first HI-stimulus but the elevated resting baseline has certainly a great deal to do with cognitive fear, which was probably denied in paper-pencil measures in terms of significance differences. Some features in the meditation technique may have facilitated higher expectancy fear expressed physiologically and in relatively higher values in state anxiety and noise estimates. PMR did perhaps the opposite as mentioned already.

Heightened heart rate expectancy – specific to multimodal meditation technique?

The meditation consisted of two major parts: 17 minutes of breathing practice by Aum-chanting (pranayama) and 13 minutes of listening to music and instruction. In detail

> ➤ listening to musical (*Raga*) recitals of Sanskrit verses by Kabhir, a mystic; then translated into English;

> ➤ instruction about visualising representations of chakras, concentrating on the centre forehead between eyebrows and „listening to the *sound within*" while

> ➤ chanting the mantras of the chakras along with visualising their symbols with colours for two minutes;

> ➤ chanting Aum for two minutes in high pitch;

> ➤ chanting *Aum* for 15 minutes in low pitch,

The literature allowed suggesting activating or alerting effects coming from all five features and here it is looked at all but the last, which will be dealt with in great detail in the next part of the discussion.

1. Becker & Shapiro (1981) found higher EEG responsivity to clicks in meditators whose techniques included concentrating on the "sound within". Pennebaker's (1982) results about *interoception* could be consistent with this: Focussing attention to internal stimuli enhances the strain of external stimulation. The instruction to concentrate on the sound within was given before the long *Aum*-chanting phase and after a phase of imagining the different "energy centres," the *chakras* to be imagined throughout the torso, neck and head.

> 'Please bring all your attention between your eyebrows and please try to listen simultaneously while singing Aum. You are calling yourself, your 'self' is listening, and try to listen in the silent moments when your Self is singing the sound from within.'

The instruction tries to focus visual attention to the centre of the forehead and simultaneously direct auditory attention to the internal environment of the body. Then: in the gaps between the *Aum* sequences, the silent moments, the subject was asked to listen intently to an internal sound, the sound within, related to *Aum*. This technique practised at least once or if desired even twice a day may have developed a similar habit of focussing attention during times of passivity as sitting in the laboratory chair[16]. Additionally: the experiment itself involved exclusively the listening modality although the subjects were not instructed to focus on the sound but to be as relaxed as possible. However, if the

---

[16] after a long period of training such attitude is likely to be developed, subjective statement of the author

meditation instruction already had conditioned this kind of interoceptive attitude, then it could have enhanced the effect of the threatening impending HI-stimulus enhanced again by passive coping and would explain both elevations of baseline and anticipation HR.

2. High pitch *Aum* chanting has an activating effect on according to a preliminary study conducted by Gore (1993) at the Indian Governments Yoga Research Department Kaivalyadham[17], Lonavla, State of Maharashtra. Marginally significant increase of HR by 6bpm was found during the high pitch recitation whereas no changes were found with low pitch recitation. Both types of *Aum*-recitation were used in our study.

3. It is not unlikely that the daily training of listening to music, to the mantra *Aum* and to their own produced sounds have sensitised the listening modality thereby increasing responsivity to stimulation: Particularly a humming sound puts the whole skull into a vibrating condition. This humming vibration could be somewhat sensitising for the cochlea. This explanation would be consistent with the fact, that in the second session the meditation group had relatively higher estimates of the compound stimulus than in the first session. The other two groups in comparison had lowered their values in the second session.

Finally, it is yearlong training with the ASDY meditation-technique, subjective experience though, that has made the author of this thesis speculate on effects of *Aum* - chanting on the viscera in the thoracic region. One can similar suggestions in the literature on *hatha* yoga on „sounding Aum and other mantras" giving a „vibro-massage to various glands and vital organs in the thoracic cavity and stimulating deeper breathing." (van Lysebeth, citation by Hewitt, p.445). It might have an impact on the heart-muscle itself. In this context it should be noted that the designer of this particular technique (També, 1982, 1998) has been successful[18] in rehabilitation of severely ill patients with coronary heart disease. Among physiotherapeutic, dietary, and ayurvedic medication measures this meditation technique is an almost compulsory common daily practice for the patients. *Aum*-chanting phases are extensive in these meditations.

Medical Science rediscovered controlled breathing

Since respiration is not primarily an autonomous system but even highly affected by voluntary control it was actually never a major player among the psychophysiological variables – as it were for example cardiovascular or electrodermal activity. As in this study it has been used therefore to control for sinus arrhythmia. However, during the last seven years, when the data acquisition forming the basis of this thesis had finished for a while, the respiratory effects on the cardiovascular system have come into the forefront of scientific scrutiny.

It was exactly the respiratory system's openness to voluntary control why investigations in controlled breathing became cutting edge of behavioural medical science research. It started with a paper on 'Continuous positive airway pressure increasing heart rate variability in congestive heart failure' (Butler, et al., 1995) since low heart rate variability as a consequence of heart failure was a marker of poor prognosis. Other papers followed on

[17] in fact one of the laboratories where Bagchi & Wenger also made their studies (see Introduction).
[18] Indian and German government awards for merits in complementary medicine, most recently for a lifestyle project at the World Exposition 2000, Hanover.

beneficial effects of controlled breathing techniques such as synchronising the respiratory-cardiovascular system due to the link between the two centres in *medulla* and *pons* of the brain stem.

Credit ought to be given to the sages of ancient India who were ingenious enough to make conscious use of the most important vital function of the human body, in order to maintain a healthy state of the human organism. They indeed drafted a system of controlled breathing techniques with specified therapeutic effects and the terms describing these techniques are almost part of the Indian day-to-day languages. *Pranayama* (from *prana* = vital force and ayama = expand) plays a primordial role in Patanjali's recommendations for achieving *Samadhi* and he perhaps did not even need to explain the techniques – so much common knowledge may those have been in his time (Hewitt, 1983, chapter on Pranayama). With help of controlled breathing techniques the yogi was supposed to connect with his soul, the *Atman* which by Vedic teaching is regarded as part of *Brahman* the highest consciousness or the creative force of nature. Interestingly, in the German language this relationship seems to be preserved by using the word *atmen* for breathing and *Atem* for breath.

So, how does all this relate to the results being discussed here and what is going to be done in the following sections? The meditation technique used in our trials to modify responsivity related to the Cardiac Defense Response consisted in its major part of a simple form of controlled breathing, namely chanting *Aum* and mantras referring to assumed „energy centres" of the body. Since we had an adaptive effect in the meditators' respiration-rate during the second experimental session possibly facilitating a recovery effect in heart rate it seems not to be foolhardy to attribute this effect to the daily respiratory training led by the taped instruction. In this context a close look will therefore be taken at the features of the chanting technique used and the immediate cognitive effects the technique had on the variable Mood consistent with results of another study using similar features of controlled breathing (Wood, 1993). The second study referred to in this context is about effects of culturally different religious recitation that gives us some idea about the central processes underlying the mood changes following controlled breathing (Bernardi, Sleight et al. 2001). Further studies (Sanderson, Yeung et al. 1996, Peng, Mietus et al., 1999) will be reported to explain why not only feelings of calm and well being can follow pranayama exercise but also of alertness and energy in some cases. Thereby these findings will help to explain the meditators' baseline-shift and anticipatory excitation of the impending stressor.

Aum-chanting practice affected breathing pattern after stressor impact

There were two more effects in physiological variables other than heart-rate, one of which was a parallel effect to SM-Group X Time differences of HR in the second session's phasic response to the repetition of HI-stimulus. (That again was a continuation of the differences in the warning sequences, SM-Group X Repetition X Session effect). Parallel to the event in the HI-stimulus repetition sequence, the meditators had reduced their respiration-rate by 1.27 cpm in contrast to an increase of 0.75 cpm in the first session while the other Groups had changes of maximally 0.27 cpm (SM-Group X Session X Repetition effect, p<0.01). A part of this effect could be accounted for by regression to the mean since the meditators had shifted their mean in the first warning sequence (see Fig. 33.3), which was part of the averaged first stimulus value (13.5, Δ=1.06 cpm). However, the Control

Group had shown a similar session shift (Δ= 0.65 cpm) and the relaxers had been at that higher initial level in the first session already.

The stark reduction in the meditators' repetition value suggested respiratory sinus-arrhythmia as a result of 4-5 weeks daily chanting. To be more precise: This phase consisted of seventeen minutes of *mantra* chanting, out of which fifteen minutes were dedicated to low pitch *Aum*. During the main 15 minutes the periods of exhalation were stretched extensively by the tape-given pattern, so that slow breathing with an average rate of 5.68 (+-1.33) breaths per minute (average measure of the experimenter's own practise over time) was induced if the guidance by the tape was followed. The long exhalation period also most likely deepened the inhalation phase.

The point being made here is, that this breathing exercise practised daily over 4 or 5 weeks may have triggered this marked change in respiration-rate when the last challenge of HI-stimulation had been experienced by the meditators. That controlled breathing practice has an effect on breathing habits is known from yoga practitioners (Bernardi, Porta et al., 2001) and in fact the rationale behind pranayama exercise is such habit changing effect as it is explained by Hewitt (1983, Chapter 6). That notion is also supported by Bernardi et al.'s study on modifications of respiratory breathing patterns in chronic heart-failure (1998). They found that the training had at least the effect of better coordination of the respiratory muscles and of the diaphragm including the facility to slow down the breathing rate, regardless of whether or not it permanently modified the spontaneous breathing habit.

Another fascinating aspect of pranayama techniques is that beneficial cognitive effects have been found earlier.

Immediate Effects on Mood and its possible underlying Central Mechanisms

Peveler & Johnston (1986), had suggested positive mood changes for both relaxation and meditation techniques and their hypothesis was confirmed in this study. PMR and ASDY-Meditation had significant effects on measures of experienced *distress, appraisal* and *arousal* assessed by the adjective-check-list. The slope difference in arousal suggested starker effects of meditation but there was no SM-Group X Training difference (p=0.21; Fig. 36.8) because of more variability in the post training values. However, there were two interesting effects at item level: meditators had reliably higher levels post meditation in the adjectives *alert* (p=0.01) and less in *sluggish* (p=0.04) than the relaxers had post PMR-training.

Cognitive Effects of Pranayama

Our findings were found to be in line with a study the effects of pranayama compared to PMR and visualisation by Wood (1993). *Pranayama (pran* = vital force, *ayama* = expand) contains a range of controlled breathing techniques and actually is integrated in most Eastern sets of meditation-practices.

The pranayama techniques investigated by Wood in a design similar to ours with repeated measurement involved a similar technique. Exercises practised in two sessions contained brief periods of relaxation and observation of the breath and mainly "physical stretching and contraction exercises together with deep breathing and forced exhalation, sometimes accompanied by humming or other vocalisation." (p.255).

The two competing methods were visualisation and progressive muscle relaxation combined with an „unspecific imagery exercise". Three groups of subjects (age range 21-71) did all three types of stress management (2 sessions of 25-30 minutes in different order). After each session the subjects were asked to rate on analogue scales their levels of *physical* and *mental energy, enthusiasm, alertness, sluggishness, sleepiness* and the degree to which they felt *calm, upset* or *nervous*. Pranayama made subjects feel reliably more *energetic* in both dimensions as well as more *enthusiastic* and *alert*. Relaxation made subjects feel reliably more *sluggish* than pranayama and reliably less *energetic*. The results of our investigation of mood-changes are similar not only because two adjectives (*alert, sluggish*) had significant differences but also because the other adjectives they had in common as *calm* and *sleepy* showed no differences at all. There was one difference though in the adjective *energetic* between the studies. We had overall differences with the meditators feeling more *energetic* ($p=0.01$) but no SM-Group X Training differences ($p=0.64$).

Wood's approach was based on the notion that the capacity of individuals to function effectively and to achieve their desired aims depends not only on their state of physical fitness. Namely it depends also on their „*perception of whether they possess the requisite levels of mental and physical energy to perform* the task in hand". (P. 254).

He therefore was interested in the question whether the perception of vitality can be reliably increased by stress management methods like relaxation, visualisation, and pranayamic exercise. He also wanted to know whether this would result in an actual increase in physical or mental energy, which is discriminated by most individuals (ibidem).

Both our Groups had relatively reduced subjective energy levels after stress management. That may indeed be a semantic problem. Wood differentiated between *physical and mental energy* levels and then pooled the answers. The author did not reveal the ratings for the two kinds separately. Since alertness clearly relates to something like mental energy we would have a *contradictio in adjecto* here, if we assumed that subjects understood the item as referring to *mental* energy. It is suggested that the adjective *energetic* in day-to-day language be actually more understood as a *physical* property. For example people think that the need or drive to move around or just to act physically, „to do something", is a sign of a high energy level. That is not the case from a yogic perspective. The capacity to act physically must be high at the same time as the capacity to be completely still. Having an urge for action, unless in reaction to challenges from the environment, can therefore be seen rather as a symptom of lack of energy as the opposite can, an overly relaxed state. By discriminating mental and physical energy from one another Wood prevented such a misunderstanding. The two energy properties were highly correlated in Wood's study after stretching and breathing exercise over half an hour. It is suggested here that application of two energy properties would have resulted in a lower correlation because our subjects were sitting still for half an hour, but given the high ratings of alertness the speculation is perhaps not too daring that mental energy would have triggered a similar result.

What could explain the increased alertness our meditators and Wood's pranayama subjects sensed? The perception of vigour is an emotional and affective state, as Wood claims, resulting from the integration at central level of a large number of physiological messages relating to the organism's physical capacity at that moment.

Studies on different variants of controlled breathing have meanwhile shed some light on those central processes initiated by the stimulus of pranayama techniques. A major central level of integration is located in *medulla* and *pons* where respiration and cardiovascular steering interact and that interaction seems to be synchronized by traditional religious recital techniques as Bernardi, Sleight et al, 2001) discovered. That is because the authors of the study suggested that increased feelings of calmness and well being found with recitals of that kind can at least in part be accounted for by the techniques under scrutiny such as Rosary Prayer or Tibetan mantra chanting (Bernardi, Sleight et al., 2002).

Physiological effects of Pranayama

Synchronisation of Respiration with the Cardiovascular System

An Italian/Polish research-group "serendipitously" found out that reciting the Rosary and a Tibetan mantra enhanced and synchronised inherent cardiovascular rhythms because the recitals reduced breathing rates to almost exactly 6 cycles per minute. At that frequency, perhaps astonishingly, is the endogenous circulatory rhythm of the human organism timed. As the authors explained in their paper healthy animals and humans show rhythmic fluctuations in blood pressure and heart rate as a result of autonomic control systems that are influenced by respiration, autonomic activation and physical activity.

A discourse about a ten-second cycle for the human blood pressure, 6 cpm accordingly, appeared already about one and a quarter of a century ago in the publications of the Viennese academy of sciences (Mayer, 1876). This endogenous circulatory rhythm is assumed to be either generated by a central nervous oscillator in the medulla or by imperfect feed back control of the slow sympathetic baroreflex and/or the fast vagal response system to respiratory changes in blood pressure. There are only good things to be said about this circulatory rhythm according to Bernardi, Sleight et al: among other things it promotes respiratory sinus arrhythmia, and consequently a slow heart rate, further the baroreflex, oxygenation of the blood and exercise tolerance. Today it is known that heart infarct patients have a lack of sympathetic heart rate variability and reduced sensitivity of their baroreceptor reflex, and that both are independently predictors of poor prognosis in heart disease.

The Rosary Prayer, a repetitive prayer form from the Roman Catholic tradition consisting of the frequent repetition of the most common prayers (Ave Maria, Lord's Prayer) was investigated in parallel with a Tibetan recital of the famous mantra sequence in Pali language which was probably „Om Mane Padme Hum".the meaning of the mantra being "Jewel in the Lotus" (The authors wrongly quoted "Om Mane Padme Om").

Six-minute recitals of the two cultural different religious verses were compared to free talking and a spontaneous breathing baseline. It was found that the recital technique, using the Latin language form, induced a breathing rate of less than 6 breaths per minute on average and so did the Tibetan recital of the Pali mantra. The studies were undertaken in

Italy, the subjects were instructed only in the Tibetan technique to repeat the mantra „with an alive, resonant voice, to listen to the sound produced, to let it flow freely"; and to pause after the end of the mantra if needed before the next cycle. The rosary prayer was tested in a condition where two subjects took over one part of the Ave Maria similar to priest and congregation in the church. Measures taken were respiration rate, heart period (the reverse of heart rate namely the averaged distance between two heart beats) for heart rate variability, systolic/diastolic blood pressure, baroreflex sensitivity and mid brain flow velocity.

By means of spectral analysis the authors found intriguing evidence for complete synchrony in oscillations of respiration rate, cardiovascular variables and mid-cerebral blood-flow. Most striking was the almost complete synchrony of respiration, heart period and systolic blood pressure as a result of the regular slow breathing rate during recitation. Spectral analysis showed that the cycles in variability of heart rate and blood pressure coincided with the respiration rate at 6cpm. In terms of frequency bands it meant that the 10th part of each of the three cycles was completed at one second or the cycles coincided at 0.1 Hz. This modulation of the cardiovascular rhythms then seemed having had an effect on the cardiovascular control mechanism in the brain stem. The arterial baroreflex sensitivity, i.e. the responsivity of the pressure sensitive receptors regulating blood pressure in the *aorta*, increased from free talking to recitation of mantra and rosary prayer.

The record of one subject suggested differences in the effects the two techniques had on heart rate: the rosary technique showed a higher average heart rate around which heart rate varied than the Tibetan mantra technique. Also the rosary amplitudes were lower than the mantra ones – both differences make sense considering the different pressures that the subjects were under. While the Tibetan technique let the subject find and follow the own pace, the rosary was practised in a dialogue, which forced each of the subjects into the pace given by the opposite recitation. The meditators of our study were in this respect more comparable to the Rosary group than to the Mantra group. Their technique was clearly activating because of the pace given by the chanting on the tape.

It seems natural that the balance of sympathetic and vagal control over the system would produce feelings of well being and harmony, which is one of the "good things" included further above. Would it not also make sense that such a state may also evoke openness for stimulation, expressed by feelings of alertness or mental energy ticked on the adjective list, which distinguished pranayama from the relaxation practitioners and thereby also higher anticipatory responsivity to a threat?

There is at last an interesting issue to be raised: Could those Sages from the Vedic times possibly have known before Mayer about this frequency? It should be mentioned in this context that not only the Tibetan Mantra has its natural roots in India. The crusaders picked the rosary up from the Arabs and those had it from the Tibetans who again had it from the Bhuddists (Lehmann, 1976, cit. Bernardi, Sleight et al. 2001) spreading out from India propagating some of the Vedic techniques removed from the cast system.

Pranayama increased Heart Rate Variability

Two more studies on effects of *controlled breathing* or *pranayama* (Sanderson, Yeung et al., 1996; Peng, Mietus et al., 1999) suggested that the breathing pattern practised along with the audiocassette not only slowed down respiration rate but also added to heart rate variability of the meditation subjects.

Heart-rate time-series were for example by Sanderson et al. coherence analysed for sinus arrhythmia on the basis of the respiration signal measured by changes of chest circumference. By means of Fourier analysis both, by their varying nature in both directions, sinusoidal signals were broken down into their components and described in terms of *amplitude, frequency* and *phase* relationship. Information about the variation of heart-rate changes over time was gained in terms of low (LF: 0.025Hz – 0.15Hz) and high frequency (HF: 0.15–0.35 Hz) bands, which covered also the range of spontaneous respiration rates. The numbers indicated the proportion of the cycle that had passed at 1 second (=1Hz), thus heart rate oscillations found at 0.2 Hz would prove a high degree of variability in heart rate. The average value for a normal respiration rate of 15 cpm described in these terms then is 0.25 Hz.

Thus it was looked for the relationship of the „natural" sinusoidal signal respiration rate measured by changes in chest circumference to a highly complex signal as heart rate changes (measured by inter-beat-intervals, the inverse of beats per minute) in both directions over longer and shorter periods of time.

The interesting thing about low and high frequency changes in heart rate in our context is that heart failure patients have a reduced rate in low frequency variability, which is a predictor of sudden death. The lack of slow changes after heart failure is seen as a paradox in the literature because they are accounted for by the sympathico-baroreceptor control in contrast to fast changes accounted for by vagal control. Thus the ratio of low and high frequency heart rate (LF/HF) is an indicator for the balance/imbalance of the two systems. The purpose of the studies was to identify the frequency both cycles of changes (oscillations) had in common or at which they covaried; in other words whether controlled breathing rates induced a form of heart rate sinus arrhythmia. The reason for that was that at the time respiration rate was mostly not controlled in studies with heart failure (see Sanderson, Yeung *et al.*, 1996 for reference).

Ten breaths enhance high frequency heart rate variability

There is a saying in German to take ten deep breaths before getting excited about something unpleasant. Folk psychology seems to be right here: Sanderson et al. found that 10 breaths taken at a minute have beneficial effects on the cardiovascular system. They studied the effects of controlled breathing conditions (10, 15 and 20cpm, 0.17; 0.25 and 0.33 Hz respectively) and posture (supine, standing) on heart rate variability in heart failure patients and normal subjects.

i.   In supine position heart rate variability is high in the high frequency band for all subjects, heart failure patients showed a reduced low frequency variability, (and indeed also if standing).

ii.   Normal subjects showed a stark increase of LF heart rate variability from supine to standing when breathing spontaneously.

iii. Normal subjects had a reversal of low and high frequency proportion at 10 cpm, controlled breathing, i.e. a very significant increase in HF variability. LF variability was markedly larger again at 20 cpm respiration rate, at 15cpm there was a slight dominance of HF. Hence spontaneous breathing (usually at about 15 cpm) produces similar results as 20 cpm controlled breathing.

iv.   For heart patients LF power increased across all conditions due to extremely reduced LF at spontaneous breathing.

Lack of LF power is a predictor for sudden death and heart failure is still the predominant killer in the western civilisation. One wonders why controlled breathing techniques are not in the headlines of the newspapers health sections at least for a couple of years as much as green vegetables are. One wonders because slow breathing becomes a habit with regular practice.

Both our Stress-Management Groups practised in a sitting position and Sanderson et al's findings should be applicable by consideration of less strain on the cardiovascular system than in a standing position. However, sitting upright has a lot in common with standing because the blood has to be pumped to the upper parts of the body and puts the body under less strain than standing, but more than lying does. So, we can assume that heart rate variability is less in sitting position (as it is in also in attention requiring tasks.)

Culturally different meditation techniques enhance low frequency heart rate variability

Peng, Mietus et al (1999) investigated two culturally different meditation techniques (Chinese and Indian) incorporating various controlled breathing techniques as different as intentional slow breathing along with visualisation and chanting.

The two techniques were

➢ Chinese Chi-technique also known as Qigong and

➢ Indian Kundalini meditation (Yogi Bhajan)

Both in a cross-legged sitting position were compared to three activities not related to meditation:

➢ Sleep of elite athletes in their pre-race period,

➢ Metronomic breathing and

➢ Spontaneous nocturnal breathing, both of healthy young adults.

Four Kundalini meditators were regarded as advanced and their measurement was taken in the laboratory. The eight subjects of the *Chi*-technique were relative beginners with 1-3 months of training and their heart-rate was measured with an ambulant device over a longer period of time including monitoring of day-today-activities. For that reason an appropriate procedure allowing ambulatory data aquisition was employed (Hilbert). The Chinese technique was practised along with taped instructions from their master who told them to breathe spontaneously while visualising the opening and closing of a perfect lotus in the stomach. The Indian technique consisted of a sequence of breathing and chanting exercises. Both meditation practises lasted for about an hour. For the end analysis the data of the meditators of both techniques were pooled and compared to the three control groups.

The results confirmed the already reported results on sinus arrhythmia induced by controlled breathing and contributed valuable information about the effects of those meditation techniques that employ pranayama.

i.   The oscillations between pre-meditation and meditation values were reliably different at within subject level, i.e. the meditation period showed extremely prominent heart rate oscillations for both kinds of meditations. For some subjects for example heart-rate varied over a 30-35 bpm range within 5 seconds. The average peak of these time series was found in the range from 0.025-0.35 Hz and coherence analysis showed that heart-rate and respiration oscillations were highly correlated (0.8) at ≈0.05Hz, which equals an extremely low respiration rate of 3 cpm. A smaller peak was also found at 0.18 Hz with 10 cpm breathing rate. The graphic displays of one chi- subject's power spectra with the two variables peaking at 0.05 Hz were almost identical in profile and structure.

ii.   Hence the pattern of heart-rate variability induced by meditation was based on *sinus-arrhythmia.*

iii.   The heart-rate oscillations of pooled meditators and control groups were reliably different in the experimental breathing phases (athletes' pre-race sleep, healthy adults' metronomic and normal sleep).

iv.   In contrast heart-rate oscillations during spontaneous breathing were not different between experimental and control groups.

The authors were happy to confirm the hypothesis that meditation is not just a measure to achieve quiescent physiological values but also an activating process. They emphasised that subjectively the subjects had experienced a profound state of deep relaxation at the same time.

There are some flaws in the study as for example regarding the control conditions: the control conditions were all in a supine position. The metronomic breathing group's respiration rate was not given. Then: respiration was an ECG derived signal and so the variables must have been correlated. A device recorded the distances of the ECG chest-electrodes from the skin, giving information about changes in chest circumference. So, this study awaits replication with better control but in the light of the other studies on controlled breathing these results can be taken into account for the discussion of our data. Thus *Fourier* analysis obviously contributed a lot to the psychophysiology of meditation as far as complex meditation techniques are concerned.

The authors noted that their Fourier frequency bands only roughly described the low and high frequency bands typically used in the literature and therefore comparison is not unproblematic. The Hilbert powers described precisely the actual power of the observed oscillations because it was calculated on the basis of one single predominant frequency. The bands used by Peng et al. therefore appeared consistently lower than the usual Fourier bands.

Conclusions

The meditation subjects of our study practised daily 17 minutes of controlled breathing at an average rate of 5.7 cycles per minute. The immediate cognitive results in the variable Mood were consistent with Wood's study about patients practising pranayama and feeling more *alert* and *energised* and less *sluggish* than practitioners of muscle relaxation. The physiological basis for this consistency has probably been revealed by three spectral analytical studies investigating the effects of controlled breathing on heart rate variability and sinus arrhythmia. Recitation techniques that control respiration rate down to 6 cpm like Rosary Prayer and Tibetan mantra chanting (5.7 cpm) increase heart rate variability in the low frequency band (0.1 Hz) and synchronise the cycles of all cardiovascular variables. Heart rate variability increases also in the low frequency band with high amplitude oscillations when subjects meditate in a cross-legged position using controlled breathing techniques such as slow breathing or chanting techniques. Controlled breathing at the higher rate of 10 cpm increases HRV more in the high frequency range of heart rate (0.16 Hz). The evidence from the reported studies therefore suggested that the meditators' heart rate variability of this study was increased too and indeed in the low frequency band, which is usually taken as an indicator of sympathicotone regulation. The activated pattern of heart rate variability is an activated one and therefore may explain changes in SCL levels of the cardiac Accelerators and the meditators increased feelings of alertness and reduced sluggishness (compared to the relaxers) as they indicated on adjective-check-lists immediately after meditation.

Given they meditated on the morning of the experiment as they were requested it is not unreasonable to assume that they were more apprehensive than the Relaxation and Control group before the second experiment and therefore had elevated resting baselines compared to the other two SM-Groups. Also their cognitive practice giving attention to the inner body-environment and the activating end-phase of high-pitch *Aum*-chanting may have increased apprehension. However, their second resting baseline, *recovery* baseline as we termed it, habituated back almost to the first session resting baseline, and they could cope well with the second stimulus set as their habituating phasic heart rate at repetition showed. Slowing down their breathing-rate in those sequences, as another repetition effect in the respiration data suggested, probably facilitated this habituating behaviour with repetition.

The meditators' were initially in the second session more „excited" than in the first session in contrast to Control and Relaxation Group. It probably is this increased excitability, due to increased heart rate variability as we know now, that could, partially at least, explain the popularity of those meditation techniques based on pranayama techniques as for example *Zen*. It does also explain popularity of Transcendental Meditation at the advanced level and therefore also the parallel features between our study and that one of Goleman & Schwartz because the *Siddhi* techniqe includes breathing and exercise practised before the usual mantra meditation. More basic pranayamic exercises are also part of a preparation phase before mantra meditation for the beginners of that technique.

4.5. Critical Reflection and Perspectives

Critical Reflection

More assessment and evaluation of respiratory data

Although this research work for a Ph.D. is more clinically oriented rather than basic research, in hindsight it would have been wise to put more emphasis on the evaluation of respiratory data given that this variable came into focus of cardiac research efforts at the time. A reliable evaluation of amplitude would not have been possible on the polygraphic records, however, a trend surely could have been indicated about influences of sinus arrhythmia.

Subjective data during experiment

One interesting result of this investigation was the between subject difference in two items (alertness and sluggishness) on the arousal scale of the adjective-check-list. This effect occurred obviously due to the pranayamic component of the multimodal meditation technique under investigation as a parallel result from a recent study on mood effects of pranayama suggested (Wood, 1994). Not to measure mood changes during the physiological experimental sessions, namely directly before and after the experiment before removing the electrodes seems to be the most serious mistake made by the author. These data could have perhaps supported the hypothesis of better recovery in the repetition periods of warning on side of the meditators. Another mistake was also made: the blood pressure data were taken after electrodes had been removed and thereby subjects had recovered from the impact of the stress experiment. Both omissions hahad to do with ethical problems on side of the author.

Non-random selection and no control over PMR practice

The other flaws of this study have already been mentioned as non-random allocation to the groups and lack of control over compliance to the demand of daily training in muscle relaxation. It would have been impossible without further resources to change the latter. The former was even more impossible to overcome because of the unusually demanding character of the meditation technique. Some people find it awkward to be asked to sing along with a tape. TM has a less embarrassing, user-friendlier secretive practice-potential. However, different people are attracted to different techniques as evidenced also by this study's failure to replicate differences between the groups on Extraversion.

Perspectives

This study treated different questions from the areas of Cardiac Defense Response, Personality and Stress Management. Perspectives for the main questions are discussed here by looking first at applied aspects of psychology. The question namely is, considering previous developments in clinical and perhaps basic research, to what extent the stress management methods of this study are of further relevance for future studies. The occupation with that question has led to some thoughts on future research interests regarding the newly flourishing research on meditation with the neuro-imaging techniques.

However, at the beginning of this final chapter it will be looked at the relevance of the original research questions of this study for the future, then, more promisingly, perspectives from single aspects developing during the course of the study will be worked out.

Research Questions of this Study

Personality and Cardiac Defense Response

Experiments with high stressor intensity are difficult to justify nowadays and not everybody may find that agreeable. Thus, no suggestions will be made for further tests of Eysenck's hypothesis on breakdown of the arousal/ activation barrier (1967) in emotional individuals. The evidence coming from Richards & Eves (1991) and this study and from the field study (Gurevich & Matveyev, 1966) may be regarded as sufficient anyway. There is no need to establish more the trivial hypothesis that highly emotional individuals will suffer most under stresses as extreme as found in wars, some may find that question unethical anyway because of its darwinistic character. Let us rather look for methods to reduce potentials for catastrophes like war instead. Academic Psychology originating in some way from war efforts (intelligence tests were first designed for American recruits) after having become predominantly an interdiscipline may dedicate some of its resources to that task by including philosophy not only for its analytical part. Approaches for that purpose have not to be searched for with great effort.

Another study on Effects of PMR on CDR related activity?

In this study we had the problem of compliance regarding PMR-training at home and the experimenter raised perhaps exaggerated reactions from the non-Accelerators by her instruction style. That possibly was the reason for failing to replicate individual differences in the warning period, which are likely to be stable over time. That poses the question whether another experiment should be undertaken to test again the hypotheses on heart rate differences in CDR-related anticipation periods and on their abolition by PMR in order to replicate the short-term study by Eves & Steptoe (1986). If any ethical committee permits such a study should be undertaken indeed. In the same investigation the other problem of this study could be solved: a fully controlled training in PMR over several weeks time with follow up measurement after 6 months as Amigo et al. (1995) did with hypertensive subjects. Then the hypothesis on direct effects of training in progressive muscle relaxation, among other methods, on cardiac hyper-reactivity could be investigated. The latter may not be a precursor of primary hypertension (Brody, Veit *et al.*, 1997) but it remains related to sudden death (Fraser, 1986, see Introduction 1.6.1).

Aspects developing from recent Literature

Neurological features related to Controlled Breathing

The training of pranayama with its effects on the cardiovascular system used in most meditation techniques seems to be efficient over a short period of time as has been already mentioned further above in context with our respiration results. Blumenthal et al. (2002)

found effects of 16 weeks of training focussing on speech pauses even after 5 years following up and speech hesitation pauses are related to controlled breathing.

Friedman (2002) suggested a cognitive model based on „neurobiological features" related to controlled breathing. He found them in literature on rehabilitation, cognitive neuroscience and, interestingly, animal behaviour. He sees for example neurobiological features suggested by correlations of rate and variability in duration of *speech hesitation pauses* (SHPs) with left and right hemispherical activity. Now, such SHPs entrain a bit of breath retention and Friedman (2000) related them to Peng et al's high amplitude oscillation patterns in those meditators practising controlled breathing. Breath retention (*khumbaka*) in the teachings of pranayama has been regarded as a phase of the controlled breathing process as important as exhalation (*rechaka*) and inhalation (*puraka*). Special emphasis has been given to it in more advanced yogic practice in order to achieve full control of the breathing process. Thereby the automatic change from excitation to inhibition of the vagus nerve regulating exhalation and inhalation is switched from "automatic to manual control" as Hewitt put it (p.73) in order to achieve an optimally functioning physiological system during meditation practice. Synchronising effects of short breath-retentions on the cardiovascular system and cognition as quoted in Friedman's notes to various journals (see below) not only confirm the wisdom of Vedic ideas regarding the importance of all three aspects of breathing. They also afford systematic research into the health promoting aspects of the various forms of yoga practice.

Short speech hesitation pauses namely are correlated to immobility in the face of stress, an increase in planning difficulty, the state of circulation (angina or hypertension) and sixfold incidence of clinical coronary heart-disease (CHD) in two normal groups of coronary-prone patients observed prospectively for ten years (Friedman, 2001; Bortfeld & Leon et al., 2001). Friedman (2000) regarded therefore the heart-rate oscillations found by Peng, Mietus et al. in context with controlled breathing in meditation practice as a „dynamic state" offering the organism „cardiovascular protection" as a process of coordination involving connectivity between distinct cortical systems. Friedman's seminal model also explains heightened responsivity with good recovery of the meditators in this study and the reference study by Goleman & Schwartz, 1976. A well functioning synchronised system will be alert and therefore responsive to stimulation and also recover quickly.

Other features next to the correlations with hemisphericity are reduced blood pressure with speech breaks about 2 seconds and beneficial effects on angina with "consciously focusing on breathing and intervening pauses". Furthermore in a 2-seconds alternation task, implying behavioural breaks, rats showed prefrontal modulation of dopamin subserving brain stem cardio-vascular control (Dreher & Guigon et al, 2002). In contrast during stress dopamine release is reduced in prefrontal cortex (Del Arco et al, 2001). Other studies on animals' behavioural breaks (entraining also breath retention) reveal reductions in serotonin neuronal activity coordinating autonomic, motor and sensory functions and modulating dopamine, which optimizes response organisation and working memory, and regulates the microvasculature implicated in slow coronary flow as a cause for coronary angina. The microvascular response to neural activity, on the other hand, is constantly delayed by about 3 seconds and is linked to the increased coherence in EEG gamma-band activity, indicating complex task processing and suggesting "effective connectivity" of distant brain areas found in learning (Buechel, Coull et al, 1999).

In this context fits a traditional "alpha wave" case study conducted by Arambula, Peper et al. (2001). They investigated with the EEG method physiological correlates of highly advanced meditation with a Japanese yoga master and, among the usual measurements, took also data from abdominal and thoracic breathing patterns. Their subject reduced his breathing pattern down to 5 breaths per minute with predominance of abdominal diaphragmatic breathing. Their data suggested a contribution of the changed breathing pattern to the development of alpha-EEG.

Finally, a study on the beneficial effects of rhythmic speech with poetry on certain *binary differential heart dynamics*, also called *musical heart* rate rhythmicity, in comparison to classical spectral analytical parameters must not be omitted here. Bettermann, v. Bonin et al. (2002) could show that that speech therapy of this kind produces alterations in heart rate dynamics particularly well with regard to the musical heart parameter, but could also appear in the spectrum of low and high frequency variability. These changes were different from those provoked by control exercises and they persisted at least for 15 minutes following training. Perhaps learning poetry by heart was not such a bad thing after all in the education system of the earlier times? That brings us to some perspectives regarding education.

Therapeutic Effects of Yogic breathing – Consequences for Education

Controlled Breathing was discovered for psychological medicine recently as has been pointed out above. One wonders why the discovery in western medicine has taken so long because a perspective for preventive medicine was available all along given by the teachings of yoga. That breathing is at the centre of yoga has also been known in Europe since the 19th century at least within the educated classes. The relevance of further research in this matter becomes even more obvious considering the results found with *chemoreflex sensitivity* and *Cheynes-Stokes* respiration as will be explained.

Yoga practitioners, probably for ages, have given anecdotical evidence for reduced chemoreflex sensitivity in comparison to non-practitioners, which shows in higher tolerance to used up air after staying in rooms with closed windows (at seminars with non-practitioners for example). This has been clinically corroborated by Spicuzza, Gabutti *et al.* (2000) by means of re-breathing manoeuvres to conditions of *isocapnic hypoxia* and *normoxic hypercapnia* performed randomly by all subjects (N=22) in three conditions: spontaneous breathing and controlled breathing at 6 and 15cpm respectively. The latter condition was the spontaneous frequency measured with the normal subjects (n=12) in the spontaneous condition. Practice of yoga breathing decreased the chemoreflex *hypoxic* and *hypercapnic* responses measured by tidal volume (= inspiration and respiration air). The effect was largely due to the slower breathing frequency that the experimental subjects exhibited spontaneously because a similar response was found also with the controls when they breathed at 6 breaths per minute in the controlled breathing condition.

The third high frequency pranayamic condition revealed that not only the slow breathing accounted for the effect because the effect should have not occurred with high frequency controlled re-breathing. However, the yogic breathers only slightly increased their tidal volume and were significantly lower in *hypoxic* condition compared to non-yogic breathers.

The experiment thus showed that the effect occurred not only to the spontaneous slow breathing frequency of the yoga subjects but to some other „yet unknown long-term effect" of yoga training.

Furthermore: Patients with heart-failure often develop irregular respiratory patterns by inhaling at different depths, a pattern known as *Cheynes-Stokes respiration*. Breathing at a controlled frequency markedly abolished the symptom and reduced respiratory instabilities. Additionally oxygen saturation was achieved at lower as well as higher frequencies. Slower breathing also improved the indirect indices of the *ventilation/perfusion* (bloodflow) *ratio* and *alveolar ventilation*, thus proving more efficient.

Reported by the same paper was a one-month of training of patients with heart-failure in a yoga-derived breathing technique, the *complete yogic breathing* as described by Hewitt (1983). It consists of slow deep breathing with pauses between the two respiratory phases – and it is a basic breathing technique learned by *hatha* yoga beginners, not an advanced technique as the name might suggest. This pranayama technique was taught for one-hour daily either in one go or split into shorter periods distributed over a day. The result was a significant increase in exercise performance and a subjective decrease of *dyspnoe* during exercise. Resting oxygen saturation increased and there were no changes in the untrained control group. One month after the training was completed the effects were still evident and the trained subjects reduced their breathing rate. Motivation also increased during the training indicating that the task appeared feasible, moreover, worthwhile from the patients' perspective.

These findings suggest more efforts into this direction of research, in particular the relationship of specific postures and types of controlled breathing should be investigated. Such combinations can be found in the vast literature on yoga postures. This literature is a meant as a contribution to preventive medicine, which is the main purpose of original *Vedic* medical (=ayurvedic) efforts.

The fact that training in controlled breathing becomes quickly habitual and the high motivation observable in high attendance of pranayama courses available on university campus suggest educational training in pranayama as a means to support a healthy lifestyle. Similar measures have already been undertaken when nutritional education became an integral part of school curricula all over the western world. Healthy lifestyles should be on the top of the list of educationalists of the technologically more developed parts of the world were the coming generations are predicted to become obese. Not everybody wants to become a jogger or fancies "working-out" in the gym.

Perhaps more studies on Meditation Oriented Lifestyles

The use of a meditation technique together with some physical exercises (stretch and controlled breathing) and a philosophical approach as cognitive component for behavioural change has become popular in segments of the wealthy western populations. The database on meditation research nine publications incorporated meditation and five specific effects of various Pranayama techniques.

Some of the following studies are highly relevant from a health-psychological point of view, some are clinical. There is a host of studies on benefits of pranayamic exercises changing levels of oxygen consumption: Fast breathing patterns increased tone, slow ones decreased it. Alternate nostril breathing facilitated hand-grip-strength in children after ten days of practice (Raghuraj, Nagarathna *et al*, 1997) and controlled breathing over two years reduced oxygen consumption per unit work without increase of blood lactate levels in athletes (Raju, Madhavi *et al*, 1994). Yardi (2001) reviewed literature on therapeutic effects of yoga on epilepsy, in particular on seizure control.

Little basic research has been done on the effects of yoga postures or movements as yet. The popularity of controlled breathing along with yoga postures is partially explained by a study by Ebert & Kuhnemann (2001). Fast and slow classical yoga breathing patterns were investigated in the effects they had on resting skeletal muscle tone. Fast pranayama increases tone, slow reduces it.

A lifestyle study has been undertaken on young participants of a meditation and yoga camp over three months in Sweden including a vegetarian diet and, of course, refraining from alcohol, caffeine and nicotine. This program has shown reduction effects on blood pressure, body mass index (BMI), serum cholesterol, and other parameters of blood analysis in pre-post program analyses (Schmidt *et al*, 1994 and 1995). A similar study was conducted over 12 weeks on 20 normotensives and 26 hypertensives with reductions in BP, body weight, serum cholesterol and triglycerids (Sachdeva, 1994).

Studies are needed on different forms of meditative lifestyles in order to provide the public with a variety of designs for such lifestyles suitable for different groups in the population (or say segments, to put it into a term of market research). Younger adults are often drawn to such lifestyles but are equally often discouraged by negative public attitudes to lifestyles linked to eastern philosophies. Efforts of psychologists to establish multicultural tolerance often stop as soon as tendencies of "mysticism" and "cult" are suspected: e.g., a mere accurate description of a meditation technique in the methodological part of a scientific investigation can be enough to blame the author for being "mystical." Academic research ought to investigate with an open mind for the pragmatism of holistic transcultural concepts for our lives in our brave, globalised new world. A paradigmatic expansion is needed in order to provide the inhabitants of the global village with choices for their execution of the right to "pursue happiness" as manifested in the American Bill of Rights, 1789. If evidence is found that certain lifestyles are more preventive of physical and mental disease then such lifestyles ought to be recommended by the scientists. Lifestyles based on mild forms of physical exercise, mental training in positive thinking and tolerance of other beliefs should be welcomed instead of being dismissed just because of deep rooted personal and/ or ideological dislike.

Palsane, Bhavasar *et al.* (1993) presented the stress-concepts of the Indian tradition and related them to modern scientific concepts. They found parallels between the western frustration-aggression hypothesis of Dollard & Miller and Freudian concepts of stress inducing potential e.g. unfulfillable (regressive) desires and the cognitive oriented stress concept of the ancient teachings. They suggested that the Indian tradition should be extensively explored with an open mind.

> "While research in Western psychology has focused on environmental events that produce stress, the Indian tradition focuses on the goals and expectancies the individual brings to the potentially stressful situation, and the avoidance of stress via internal control. The two approaches are likely to prove complementary to each other." (p.15).

The potential „power of the mind" is now locked away in the placebo variable to keep it under control. Research ought to look at it as an experimental variable instead as it has for example been done by sport psychologists with dissociative and associative thinking (Couture, Singh *et al*, 1994).

Neurological studies on meditation as a complex Cognitive Stimulus

Another perspective opens up for meditation research following the tradition of brain research in this matter. Today there are more experienced meditators available for laboratory testing than in the seventies and that facilitates basic research into brain functions of this particular population living a certain professional yogic lifestyle in its purpose different from the subject of lifestyle-studies mentioned above.

Lehmann, Faber et al. (2001) took advantage of a Tibetan Lama's proficient visualization-techniques used for inducing different states of consciousness. The images gained from visual and verbalization tasks were found neuroanatomically correct. Neuroimages of self-induced dissolution and reconstitution of the experience of the Self were documented and discussed in neurological and clinical contexts. Advanced meditators will perhaps become another popular group of subjects perhaps as a second kind of control group for stroke patients? That is suggested because such subjects are less exposed to the usual stresses of daily life and it's counterbalancing agents like drugs and alcohol. The picture about "normal" brain processes would perhaps be more complete.

Another brain study with functional magnetic resonance imaging technique, astonishingly, was presented on transcendental meditation by Lazar, Bush et al. (2000) with Herbert Benson, one of the "inventors" of the relaxation response, featuring as last author. They had trained TM meditators to meditate along with the noise generating imaging machine that in itself seems an indicator of some advanced stage the subjects must have had achieved. Group averaged data of the five subjects indicated that TM meditation activated prefrontal and parietal cortex and midbrain structures, neural structures involved in attention and control of the autonomic nervous system. Their aim was to show correlates of the relaxation response (see Introduction).

Another, calmer but invasive technique was used by Newberg, Alavi et al. (2001) to elucidate connections between different brain areas elicited by a complex cognitive function such as a Tantric meditation technique practised by seven experienced practitioners of Buddhist Tantric meditation. The task was performed with single positron emission computer tomography (SPECT), i.e. the meditators were connected to an intravenous tube and before they started their meditation a radio-active isotope was injected as well as during their peak meditative state which they signalised to the experimenter. Baseline resting comparison with post meditation images provided by the SPECT camera brought interesting results about some neurophysiological correlates of a complex meditation form: The images revealed increased activity in the prefrontal lobes with a simultaneous trend of decreased activity in the posterior parietal lobes, an interaction known from subjects performing visual spatial tasks. High concentration of attention as demanded in an active technique explain high frontal lobe activity and also a compensatory decrease in the parietal lobes, where the sense of space and time has been located in the literature. However, this decrease was not significant and thereby not as clear as predicted by the authors.

Another prediction was contradicted by the data: the authors expected a decrease of sensomotor activity because of the inactive posture the meditators had taken during the experiment. On the contrary an increased level of activity was shown in the tomogram. The authors speculated on two possible confounding factors: A degree of activity to maintain the sitting posture and visual input from the internal images generated during this type of meditation. These speculations seem not overwhelming unless the images would include movements but usually in Tibetan meditation static Buddhas of different varieties are visualised. Unfortunately the content of the features of the complex meditation technique has not been presented. However, these hypotheses should be tested to clarify this unexpected result.

The authors also found activation of the midbrain (limbic system, hippocampus) suggesting autonomous activity during meditation and the activating character of advanced meditation practice.

While, as expected, cerebellum, superior frontal and occipital areas whose functions were not related to practice of meditation were not found activated, the SPECT image showed the *thalamus* with significantly increased activation. This result was explained by the major cortical and subcortical relay function this most important nucleus has. Responsible, according to the authors, were the "cognitive and affective responses" this type of meditation elicits in the practitioners.

This explanation makes perfect sense if we consider meditation features like visualisation and recitals being part of Tantric meditation techniques but which unfortunately did the authors not present. However, the discussed activation patterns reflected the meditators' peak of their practice and at that point no practice takes place anymore as every experienced meditator will know, and as the authors should know. Those practices are down to achieve those peaks and therefore the active character of meditation techniques does not confound those activation patterns and rejects the hypothesis of meditational states being quiescent, even comatose states of consciousness. The authors discussed their results in a very uncontroversial way it seems. In the light of these findings the activated pattern found in the EEG of the most advanced subject does also not look so artefactual anymore (Das & Gastaut, 1955; see EEG review, Introduction) as it was suggested by reviewers 40 years or so ago.

Two other results were of particular interest for the authors, and this thesis finishes with them. The group of expert meditators had a significant different laterality of their thalamus compared to the non-meditating control subjects, a finding whose potential functional meaning was not revealed in the article. Was this individual difference a consequence of yearlong practice or was it a predisposition for something like mystical experience is the question for future research tasks. If this difference is an effect of continuous meditation practice this would confirm neurologically behavioural changes in how information is processed by meditators which is a declared aim of long-term, spiritually oriented meditators. If it is a personality feature then the finding gives future scientists, educationalists and clinicians the responsibility to give spiritual efforts a legitimate place in the cannon of leisure and lifestyle activities.

References

Abrahams, V.C., Hilton, S.M. & Zbrozyna, A. (1960): Active Muscle Vasodilatation produced by stimulation of the brain stem: Its significance in the defense reaction. *Journal of Physiology* (London), 154, 491-513.

Adams, D., Baccelli, G., Mancia, G. & Zanchetti, A. (1971): Relation of cardiovascular changes in fighting to emotion and exercise. *Journal of Physiology* (London), *212*, 321-335.

Amigo, I., Gonzalez, A. & Herrera, J. (1997): Comparison of physical exercise and muscle relaxation training in the treatment of mild hypertension. *Stress Medicine, 13 (1), 59-65.*

Anand, B.K., China, G.S. & Singh, B. (1961): Some Aspects of encephalographic Studies in Yogis, *Electroencephalography and. Clinical Neurophysiology*, 13, .pp 452-456, reprint. In *Altered States of Consciousness*, revised and updated 1990[3] (ed. C. Tart), San Francisco, 596- 599.

Arambula, P., Peper, E., Kawakami, M. & Gibney, K.H. (2001): The Physiological Correlates of Kundalini Yoga Meditation: A Study of a Yoga Master. *Applied Psychophysiology and Biofeedback, 26, 2, 147-153.*

Austin, James H. (1998): Zen and the Brain: toward an understanding of meditation and consciousness. Massachusetts, Institute of Technology.

Bagchi, B.K. & Wenger, M.A. (1957): Electrophysiological correlates of some yogic exercises. *Electroencephalography and Clinical Neurophysiology,* Supplement 7. 132-149/

Banquet, J.P. (1973): Spectral Analysis of the EEG in Meditation. *Electroencephalography and Clinical Neurophysiology, 35, 143-151.*

Becker, D.E.& Shapiro, D. (1981): Physiological Responses to Clicks during Zen, Yoga and TM Meditation, *Psychophysiology* 18, 6, 694-699.

Beiman, I., Israel, E. & Johnson, S.A. (1978): During- and post-training effects of live and taped extended progressive relaxation, self-relaxation and electromyogram-feedback. *Journal of consulting & clinical Psychology, 46, 314-321.*

Benson, H. & Friedman, R. (1985): A rebuttal to the conclusions of David S. Holmes's article: „Meditation and somatic arousal reduction". *American Psychologist*, 40, 725-728.

Benson, H. & Wallace, R.K. (1972): Decreased Blood pressure in hypertensive subjects who practice meditation. *Circulation*, Supplement 2, 45, 516.

Benson, H., Beary, J.F. & Carol, M.P. (1974): The relaxation response. *Psychiatry, 37, 37-46.*

Bernardi, L., Porta, C., Gabutti, A., Spicuzza, L. & Sleight, P. (2001): Modulatory effects of respiration (Review Article). *Autonomic Neuroscience: Basic and Clinical*, 90, 47-56.

Bernardi, L., Sleight, P., Bandinelli, G, Cencetti, S., Fattorini,L., Wdowczyc-Szulc & Lagi, A. (2001): Effect of rosary prayer and yoga mantras on autonomic cardio-vascular rhythms: comparative study. *British Medical Journal, 323, 1446-49.*

Bernardi, L., Spadaccini, G., Bellwon, J., Hajric, R., Roskamm, H.& Frey, A.W. (1998): Effect of breathing rate on oxygen saturation and exercise performance in chronic heart failure. *Lancet. 351,: 1308- 1311.*

Bernstein, D. & Borkovec, T.D. (1973): Progressive Muscle Relaxation Training. Research Press, Illinois.

Bettermann, H., v. Bonin, D., Fruehwirt, M., Cysarz, D., & Moser, M. (2002): Effects of speech therapy with poetry on heart rate rhythmicity and cardiorespiratory coordination. *International Journal of Cardiology, 84, 1, 77-88.*

Birbaumer, N. &. Schmidt, R. F (1997): Wachen, Aufmerksamkeit und Schlafen. In *Physiologie des Menschen*(eds R. Schmidt & G. Thews), Berlin, Heidelberg, New York: Springer, 141-154.

Blackwell, B., Hanenson, I.B., Bloomfield, S., Magenheim, H.G., Gartside, P., Nidich, S., Robinson, A. & Zigler, R. (1976): Transcendental Meditation in hypertension: individual response patterns. *Lancet, 1, 223-226.*

Blanchard, E.B., McCoy, G.C.,Wittrock, D., Musso, A. *et al.* (1988): A controlled comparison of thermal biofeedback and relaxation training in the treatment of essential hypertension: II. Effects on cardiovascular reactivity. *Health Psychology, 7 (1), 19-33.*

Blumenthal, J.A., Babyak, M., Wei, J., O'Connor, C., Waugh, R., Eisenstein, E., Mark, D., Sherwood, A., Woodley, P.S., Irwin, R.J. & Reed, G. (2002): Usefulness of psycho-social training of mental stress-induced myocardial ischemia in men. *American Journal of Cardiology*, 2002, 89, 164-168.

Borkovec, T.D. & Sides, J.K. (1979): Critical Procedural variables related to the physiological effects of Progressive Relaxation: a review. *Behaviour, Research and Therapy,* 17, pp .119-25.

Boswell, P.C., Murray, E.J. (1979): Effects of Meditation on psychological and physiological measures of anxiety. *Journal of Consulting and Clinical Psychology, 47, 606-607.*

Brandt, K. (1973): The effects of relaxation training with analogue HR feedback on basal levels of arousal and response to aversive tones in groups selected according to Fear Survey scores. *Psychophysiology, 11, 242* (Abstract).

Brod, J., Fencl, V.S., Hejl, Z. & Jirka, J. (1959): Circulatory changes underlying blood pressure elevation during acute emotional stress (mental arithmetic) in normotensive and hypertensive subjects. *Clinical Science*, 18, 269-279.

Brody, S.; Veit, R.; Rau, H., (1996): Neuroticism but not cardiovascular stress reactivity is associated with less longitudinal blood pressure increase. *Personality and Individual Differences, 20 (3), 375-380.*

Brody, S.; Veit, R.; Rau, H., (1997): Lie scores are associated with less cardiovascular reactivity to baroreceptor stimulation and to mental arithmetic stress. *Personality and Individual Differences, 22 (3), 677-681.*

Buechel, C., Coull, J.T., Friston, K.J., (1999): The predictive value of changes in effective connectivity for human learning. *Science*, 283, 1538-41.

Busse, R. (1997): Gefässystem und Kreislaufregulation. In *Physiologie des Menschen (eds R. Schmidt & G. Thews), 498-564,* Berlin, Heidelberg, New York: Springer.

Butler, G.C., Naughton, T., Rahman, M.A., Bradley, T.,D. & Floras, J.S. (1995): Continuous Positive Airway Pressure increases Heart Rate Variability in Congestive Heart Failure. *Journal of American Cardiology, 25, 3, 672-679.*

Cannon, W.B. (1915): Bodily changes in pain, hunger, fear and rage, an account of recent research into the function of emotional excitement. New York & London: Appleton.

Carlson, N.R. (1991[4]): Physiology of Behavior, Boston, Allyn & Bacon.

Collins, J.A., & Rice, V.H. (1997): Effects of intervention in phase II cardiac rehabilitation: Replications and extensions. *Heart & Lung, 26, (1), 31-44.*

Corby, J.C., Roth, W.T., Zarcone, V.P. & Kopell, B.S. (1978): Psychophysiological Correlates of the Practice of Tantric Yoga Meditation, *Arch. Gen. Psychiatry, 35:* 571 - 577.

Couture, R.; Singh, M.; Lee, W.; Chahal, P; et al. (1994): The effect of mental training on the performance of military endurance tasks in the Canadian infantry (Abstract). *International Journal of Sport Psychology, 25(2), 144-157.*

Craske, M.G. & Rachman, S.J. (1987): Return of fear: Perceived skill and heart-rate responsivity. *British Jouranl of Clinical Psychology, 26 (3), 187-199.*

Cruickshank, P.J. (1984): A stress and arousal mood scale for low vocabulary subjects: a re-working of McKay et al. *British Journal of Psychology , 75, 89-94.*

Curtis, W.D. & Wessberg, H.W. (1975): A comparison of heart rate, respiration , and galvanic skin response among meditators, relaxers and controls. *Journal of Altered States of Consciousness, 2, 319-324.*

Das N.N. & Gastaut, H. (1955): Variations de l´áctivite eléctrique du cerveau, du coeur et des muscles squelettiques au cours de la meditation et de l´ecstase yogique, *EEG Clin. Neurophys.*, 6, (suppl.) 211 - 219.

References

Daum, I. & Schugens, M. (1986): The Strelau Temperament Inventory (STI): preliminary results in a West-German sample. *Personality & Individual Differences, 7, 509-517.*

Davidson, R. J. & Schwartz, G., E. (1976): Psychobiology of relaxation and related states. In *Behavior Modification and Control of Physiological Activity* (ed. D. Mostofsky), N.J.: Prentice-Hall, Englewood Cliffs.

Davis, R.C. (1948): Motor effects of strong auditory stimuli. *Journal of Experimental Psychology, 38, 257-275.*

Del Arco, A. & Mora, F. (2001): Dopamine release in the prefrontal cortex during stress is reduced by the local activation of glutamate receptors. *Brain Research Bulletin, 56, 125-130.*

Delman, R. & Johnson, H. (1976): Biofeedback and progressive muscle relaxation: a comparison of psychophysiological effects. *Psychophysiology, 13, 181.*

Delmonte M M. (1987b): Personality and Meditation. In: *The Psychology of Meditation, (ed. M. West)* 118 - 134, Clarendon Press, Oxford.

Delmonte, M. (1987a): Meditation: contemporary theoretical approaches. In: *The Psychology of Meditation, (ed. M. West) 39 - 53, Clarendon Press, Oxford*

Delmonte, M. M. (1984): Physiological concomitants of meditation practice, Review, *Int. Journal of eclectic Psychotherapy, 31 (4), 23 - 26.*

Delmonte, M.M. (1980): Personality characteristics and regularity of meditation. *Psychological Reports,* 46, 703-12.

Delmonte, M.M. (1988): Personality Correlates of Meditation Practice, Frequency and Dropout in an Outpatient Population. *Journal of Behavioural Medicine,* 11, 6, 593-597.

Dillbeck, M. (1977): The effect of the transcendental meditation technique on anxiety level. *Journal of Clinical Psychology,* 33, 1076-78.

Dreher, J., Guignon, E. Bernard, Y. (2002): A model of prefrontal cortex dopaminergic modulation during the delayed alternation task. *Journal of Cognitive Neuroscience, 14, 6, 853-865.*

Ebert, D. & Kuhnemann, B. (2001): Breathing pattern influences the resting innervation tone of skeletal muscles. Klinische Neurophysiologie, 32, 1, pp.30-37.

Eckberg, D.L. (1983): Human sinus arrhythmia as an index of vagal cardiac outflow. *Journal of Applied Physiology, 54, 961-966.*

Elliott, R. (1972): The significance of the heart rate for behavior: A critique of Lacey's hypothesis. *Journal of Personality and Social Psychology, 22, 398-409.*

Endler, N.S. & Magnusson, D. (1976): Toward an interactional psychology of personality. *Psychological Bulletin, 83, 956-974.*

References

English, E.H. & Baker, T.B. (1983): Relaxation Training and cardiovascular response to experimental stressors, *Health Psychology*, 2 (3) 239 - 259.

Eppinger, H. & Hess, L. (1910): Die Vagotonie. Berlin, Springer.

Eves, & Gruzelier, J.H. (1987): Individual differences in vascular components of the defensive response, *Journal of Psychophysiology*, 1,161-172.

Eves, F. F. & Gruzelier, J. H. (1984): Individual Differences in the Cardiac Response to High Intensity Auditory Stimulation, *Psychophysiology, 21, 342 - 352.*

Eves, F. F., Blizard, B. Levey, A. & Martin, I. (1990): Cardiac reactions to passive stimulation in twins. In *European Perspectives in psychology* (eds. Arenth, P.J.D., Seargent, J.A. & Takens, R.J.), 443-457. Chichester: John Wiley.

Eves, F.F. & Steptoe, A. (1986): Modification of reactivity associated with the defensive response. Paper presented at the 13th annual meeting of the Psychophysiology Society, December 1985, London. *Journal of Psychophysiology, Conference report,* (Abstract).

Eves, F.F. & Steptoe, A. (1986): Relaxation modifies reactivity associated with the fight/flight response. Paper presented at the satellite symposium on Applied Psychophysiology in Hypertension at the 11th scientific meeting of the International Society for Hypertension, Bonn.

Eves, F.F. (1985): Individual differences in cardiovascular adjustment elicited by high intensity auditory stimulation in humans. Unpublished Ph.D. thesis, University of London.

Ewald, C.A. (1877): [Über die Veränderungen der kleinen Blutgefässe in der Bright'schen Krankheit und den damit verbundenen Theorien.] On the changes in small blood vessels in Bright's disease and on the associated theories. *Virchow's Arch.,* 71, 453-499.

Eysenck, H.J. & Eysenck, M.W., (1985): Personality and Individual Differences, Plenum Press, New York and London.

Eysenck, H.J. & Eysenck, S.B.G. (1963): EPI, Form B. Hodder & Stoughton London.

Eysenck, H.J. (1967): The Biological Basis of Personality, Charles C. Thomas, USA.

Eysenck, H.J. (1987): Arousal and Personality: The Origins of a Theory. In *Personality, Dimensions and Arousal* (eds. J. Strelau, & H.J. Eysenck) New York.

Fahrenberg, J. (1987): Concepts of Activation and Arousal in the Theory of Emotionality (Neuroticism): A Multivariate Conceptualization. In *Personality Dimensions and Arousal* (eds. J. Strelau, & H.J Eysenck) New York.

Fahrenberg, J. (1991): Psychophysiology of Neuroticism and Anxiety. In: *Handbook of Individual Differences: Biological Perspectives* (eds. Gale, A. & Eysenck, M.W.) Chichester.

References

Fenwick, P. (1969): Computeranalysis of the EEG during mantra meditation. *Paper presented at a conference on the effects of meditation , concentration and attention on the EEG.* University of Marseilles (as cited by Fenwick, 1987).

Fenwick, P. (1987): Meditation and the EEG. In *The Psychology of Meditation* (M.West ed.), p 104-117, Clarendon Press, Oxford.

Folkow, B. (1982): Physiological Aspects of Primary Hypertension. *Physiological Review,* 62, 347-479.

Folkow, B. (1990): „Structural Factor" in Primary and Secondary Hypertension. In: *Hypertension,* 16, (1), 89-101.

Forsyth, R.(1971): Regional bloodflow changes during 72 hour avoidance schedules in monkeys. *Science,* 173, 546-548.

Fowles, D.C. (1982): Heart-rate as index of anxiety. In *Perspectives in cardiovascular psychophysiology (eds. J. Caccioppo, & R. Petty).* The Guilford Press, New York.

Fowles, D.C., Christie, M.J., Edelberg, R., Grings, W.W., Lykken, D.T. & Venables, P.H. (1981): Publication recommendations for electrodermal measurements. *Psychophysiology*, 18, 232-239.

Fraser, G. (1986): Preventive Cardiology, New York, Oxford University Press, Chapter: The Epidemiology of Sudden Death, 195-206.

Friedman, E.H. & Coats, A.J. (2000): Neurobiology of exaggerated heart rate oscillations during two meditative techniques. *International Journal of Cardiology* 73, 199.

Friedman, E.H. (1999): Neurobiology of respiratory-pattern training in congestive heart failure (letter). *European Heart Journal, 20, 1052-53.*

Friedman, E.H. (2001): Socio-economic status and ischemic stroke (letter). *Stroke 32, 2725.*

Friedman, E.H. (2002): Neurobiology of Psychosocial Treatment of Mental Myocardial Ischemia in Men. *American Journal of Cardiology, 90, 1.*

Geen, R. (1984): Preferred stimulation levels in introverts and extraverts: effects on arousal and performance. *Journal of Personality and Social Psychology,* 46, 1303-1312.

Gilbert, G.S., Parker, J.C. & Claiborn, C.D. (1978): Differential mood changes in alcoholics as a function of anxiety-management strategies (Abstract). *Journal of Clinical Psychology,* 34, 229-232.

Goleman, D.J. & Schwartz, G.E. (1976): Meditation as an intervention in stress reactivity, *Journal of Consulting and Clinical Psychology,* 44, 456 - 466.

Gore, M.M. (1991): Anatomy and Physiology of Yoga Practices. B.M. Gore at post Kaivalyadhama, Lonavla, PIN 410 403 District Pune, India.

References

Graham, F.K. & Slaby, D.A. (1973): Differential heart-rate changes to equally intense white noise and tone. *Psychophysiology,* 10, 4 347-362.

Graham, F.K. & Clifton, R.K. (1966): Heart rate change as a component of the orienting response. *Psychological. Bulletin,* 65, 305-320.

Graham, F.K. (1979): Distinguishing among Orienting, Defense and Startle Reflexes. In *The Orienting Reflex in Humans,* (eds. H.D. Kimmel, E.G. van Olst & J.H. Orlebeke), 137 –167, Hillsdale, N.J., Lawrence.

Graham, F.K., (1975): The more or less startling effects of weak prestimulation. *Psychophysiology, 12, 238-248.*

Gray. J.A. (1964): Strength of the nervous system and levels of arousal: a re-interpretation. In: *Gray, J.A. (Ed.), Pavlov's Typology, Oxford: Pergamon.*

Gray. J.A. (1972): The physiological nature of introversion-*Extraversion*: a modification of Eysenck's theory. In *Biological bases of individual behaviour* (eds. V.D. Nebylitsyn, & J.A. Gray), London, Academic Press.

Green, K., Beiman, I., Webster, J., Holliday, P. & Rosmarin, D. (1977): A controlled comparison of progressive relaxation training and self-relaxation on measures of tonic physiological arousal and phasic response to fearful stimuli. *Paper presented to the 23rd Annual Meeting of the Southeastern Psychological Association, Florida.*

Gurevich, K.M. (1966): Professional fitness and basic nervous system properties. Nauka, Moscow (in Russian, cited as in Strelau 1983).

Hays, W.L. (1981): Statistics (3rd edition). New York: Holt, Rinehart & Winston.

Heistad, D. & Abboud, F. (1974): Factors that influence Bloodflow in Skeletal Muscle and Skin. *Anesthesiology* 41, 2, 139-156.

Hess, W.R. (1949): Das Zwischenhirn. Schwade & Co. Basel.

Hilton, S.M. (1963): Inhibition of baroreceptor reflexes on hypothalamic stimulation. *Journal of Physiology (London), 165, 56-57.*

Hirschman, R. & Favaro, L. (1980): Individual differences in imagery vividness and voluntary heart-rate control. *Personality & Individual Differences,* 1, 129-133.

Hochberg, J.E., Triebel, W., & Seaman, G. (1951): Color adaptation under conditions of homogenous visual stimulation (Ganzfeld). *Journal of Experimental Psychology*, 41, 153-159).

Holmes, D. S. (1984): Meditation and somatic arousal reduction:- a review of the experimental evidence, *American Psychologist* 39, 1-10.

Holmes, D. S. (1985): To meditate or to simply rest, the answer is rest. *American Psychologist, 40, 728-31.*

References

Holmes, D. S. (1987): The Influence of meditation versus rest on physiological arousal: a second examination. In *The Psychology of Meditation (ed. M. West)* 81 - 103, Clarendon Press, Oxford.

Holmes, D.H., Solomon, S., Cappo, B.M. & Greenberg, J.L. (1983): Effects of transcendental meditation versus resting on physiological and subjective arousal. *Journal of Personality and Social Psychology*, 44, 1245-1252.

Honderich, T., *ed* (1995): The Oxford Companion to Philosophy. Oxford University Press.

Howell, D. C. (1992): *Statistical Methods for Psychology - 3rd edition*. Belmont, CA, Duxbury Press.

Jamner, L.D. & Schwartz, G.E. (1986): Self-deception predicts self report and endurance of pain. *Psychosomatic Medicine, 48, 211-223.*

Jamner, L.D., Schwartz, G.E. & Leigh, H. (1988): The relationship between repressive and defensive coping styles and monocyte, eosinophile, and serum glucose levels: Support for the opioid peptide hypothesis of repression. *Psychosomatic Medicine, 50, 567-575.*

Jänig, W. (1997): Vegetatives Nervensystem. In *Physiologie des Menschen* (eds R. Schmidt & G. Thews), Berlin, Springer, 340-369.

Jevening, R., Wallace, R.K. & Beidebach, M. (1992): The Physiology of Meditation: A Review. A Wakeful Hypometabolic Integrated Response. *Neuroscience and Biobehavioral Reviews. 16, 415-424.*

Jorgensen, R.S. & Houston, B.K. (1986): Family history of hypertension, personality patterns, and cardiovascular reactivity to stress. *Psychosomatic Medicine, 48, 102-117.*

Kanas, N. & Horowitz, M.J. (1977): Reactions of TM-meditators and non-meditators to stress-films: a comparative study. *Archives of General Psychiatry*, 34, 1431-6.

Kasamatsu, A. & Hirai, T. (1966): An Electroencephalographic Study on the Zen Meditation (Zazen), *Folio Psychiat.& Neurolog. Japonica, 20, 1966, 315-336*, reprinted in: *Altered States of consciousness, revised and updated 1990^3* (ed. C. Tart), 581-595, San Francisco: Harper & Collins.

Kiecolt-Glaser, J.K. & Greenberg, B. (1983): On the use of physiological measures in assertion research. *Journal of Behavioral Assessment, 5, 97-109.*

Kiefer, D. (1985): EEG alpha feedback and subjective states of consciousness. A subject's introspective overview. In *Frontiers of Consciousness*, J. White. (*ed.*) New York, Julian Press, 94-113.

Kiefer, D. (1985): EEG alpha feedback and subjective states of consciousness. A subjects introspective overview. In: *Frontiers of Consciousness*, ed. J.White. New York, Julian Press, pp. 94-113.

Kirsch, I. & Henry, D. (1979): Self- Desensitization and Meditation in the reduction of public speaking anxiety. *Journal of Consulting and Clinical Psychology,* 47, 536 - 541.

Kline, J.P., Schwartz, G.E., Fitzpatrick, D.F. & Hendricks, S.E. (1993): Defensive-ness, Anxiety and the amplitude / intensity function of auditory-evoked potentials. *International Journal of Psychophysiology, 15, 7-14.*

Lacey, J. (1972): Some Cardiovascular Correlates of Sensorimotor Behavior: Examples of Visceral Afferent Feedback? In *Limbic System Mechanisms and Autonomic Function* (ed. C. Hockman), Illinois, Thomas, 175-196.

Lacey, J. I. & Lacey, B. C. (1974): On heart rate responses and behavior: A reply to Elliott. *Journal of Personality and Social Psychology, 30, 1-18.*

Landis, C. & Hunt, W.A. (1939): The startle pattern, New York, Academic Press.

Lazar, S.W., Bush, G., Gollub, R.L., Fricchione, G.L., Khalsa, G., & Benson, H. (2000): Functional Brain mapping of the relaxation response and meditation. *NeuroReport, 11, 7, 1581-85.*

Lazarus, R.S. & Averill, J.R. (1972): Emotion and Cognition: With special reference to anxiety. *In C.D. Spielberger (Ed.), Anxiety: Current trends in theory and research.* New York: Academic Press.

Lehmann, D., Beeler, G.W., & Fender, D.H. (1967): EEG-Responses during the observation of stabilized and normal retinal images. *Electroencephalography and Clinical Neurophysiology*, 22, 136-142.

Lehmann, D., Faber, P.L., Achermann, P., Jeanmonod, D., Gianotti, L.R. & Pizzagalli, D. (2001): Brain sources of EEG gamma frequency during volitionally meditation-induced, altered states of consciousness, and experience of the self. *Psychiatry Research: Neuroimaging, 108, 2, 111-121.*

Lehmann, J. (1976): Die Kreuzfahrer [The Crusaders]. Munich, Bertelsmann, (cited as in Bernardi, Sleight et al.).

Lehrer, P.M. (1982): How to relax and how not to relax: A Re-evaluation of the work of Edmund Jacobson. *Behavioral Research and Therapy,* 20, 417-428.

Lehrer, P.M., Batey, D., Woolfolk, R., Remde, A. & Garlick, T. (1988): The Effect of Repeated Tense-Release Sequences on EMG and Self-Report of Muscle Tension: An Evaluation of Jacobsonian and Post-Jacobsonian Assumptions About Progressive Relaxation.

Lehrer, P.M., Schoickett, S., Carrington, P. & Woolfolk, R.L. (1980): Psychophysio-logical and Cognitive Responses to stressful stimuli in subjects practising progressive muscle relaxation and clinically standardized meditation. *Behavior, Research and Therapy, 18,* 293-303.

Lehrer, P.M., Woolfolk, R.L., Rooney, A. J., McCann, B. & Carrington, P., (1983): Progressive Relaxation and Meditation - A Study of Psychophysiological and Therapeutic Differences between two Techniques, *Behavioral Research Therapy, 21, No 6, 651-622.*

Libby, W., Lacey, B., & Lacey, J. (1973): Pupillary and cardiac activity during visual attention. *Psychophysiology, 10, 270-294.*

Linden, W. (1971): Practising of meditation by school children and their levels of field-dependence-independence, test anxiety and reading achievement. *Journal of Consulting and Clinical Psychology,* 41, 139-143.

Lisander, B. (1970): Factors influencing the autonomic component of the defense reaction. Acta Physiologica Scandinavica, Supplement 351, 1-42.

Mathews, A. & Tata, P. (1986): Attentional bias in emotional disorders. *Journal of abnormal Pscyhology, 95 (1), 15-20.*

Matveyev, V.F. (1965): Psychological manifestation of the basic properties of the nervous system in power plant operators under condition of simulated damage. In B.M. Teplov, ed., *Typological features of higher nervous activity in man.* Vol. 4, Prosveshcheniye, Moscow (in Russian, cited as in Strelau, 1983).

Mayer, S. (1876): Studien zur Physiologie des Herzens und der Blutgefaesse. 6. Abhandlung: ∞ber spontae Blutdruckschwankungen. [Studies on the physiology of the heart and the bloodvessels. 6th Discourse on fluctuations in bloodpressure.] Sitz der Akademie der Wissenschaften, Wien, Mathe-Naturwiss., Klin. Anat., 74: 281 – 307.

Michaels, R.R., Huber, M.J. & McCann (1976): Evaluation of Transcendental Meditation as Method of Reducing Stress. *Science* 192, 1242-1244.

Miltner, W.H.R., Braun, C., Arnold, M., Witte, H. & Taub, E. (1999): Coherence of gamma-band EEG activity as basis for associative learning. Nature, 397, 434-436.

Mischel, W. & Peake, P.K. (1983): Some facets of consistency: Replies to Epstein, Funder, and Bem. *Psychological Review, 90, 394-402.*

Mischel, W. (1968): *Personality and Assessment.* New York: Wiley.

Morse, D.R., Martin, S., Fuerst, M.L., & Dubin, L.L. (1977): A physiological and subjective evaluation of meditation, hypnosis and relaxation. *Psychosomatic Medicine, 39, 304-324.*

Moruzzi,G. & Magoun, H. (1949): Brainstem reticular formation and activation of the EEG. Electroencephalography & Clinical Neurophysiology, 1, 455-473.

Naranjo, C. (1971): Meditation: Its Spirit and Techniques. In *On the Psychology of Meditation (eds C. Naranjo & R. Ornstein)* 3-132, Allen & Unwin, London

Newberg, A., Alavi, A., Baime, M., Pourdehnad, M., Santanna, J. & d'Aquili, E. (2001): The measurement of regional cerebral bloodflow during the complex cognitive task of meditation: a preliminary SPECT study. Psychiatry Research-Neuroimaging, 106, 2, 113-122.

Obrist, P. (1976): Presidential Address, 1975, The Cardiovascular-Behavioural Interaction – As it Appears Today, *Psychophysiology, 13, 95-107.*

Obrist, P. (1982): Cardiac-Behavioural interactions: a critical appraisal. In *Perspectives in cardiovascular psychophysiology (eds. Caccioppo, J. & Petty, R.), New York, The Guilford Press, 265-295.*

Obrist, P.(1981): Cardiovascular Psychophysiology, New York, Plenum.

Obrist, P.A., Webb, R.A., Sutterer, J.R. & Howard, J.L. (1970): Cardiac deceleration and reaction time: An evaluation of two hypotheses. *Psychophysiology, 6, 695-706.*

Orlebeke, J.F. & Feij, J.A. (1979): The Orienting reflex as a personality correlate. In *The Orienting Reflex in Humans* (eds. H.D.Kimmel, E.H. van Olst, & J.F. Orlebeke) Erlbaum, Hillsdale. N.J.

Ornstein, R.E. (1972): The Techniques of Meditation and Their Implications for Modern Psychology. In *On the Psychology of Meditation* (eds. C. Naranjo & R. Ornstein) 137-233, London, Allen & Unwin.

Pagano, R. & Warrenburg, S. (1983): Meditation: In search of a unique effect. In *Consciousness and Self Regulation* (eds R. Davidson, G. Schwartz & D. Shapiro), New York, Plenum Press, 3, 153- 205.

Palsane, M.N., Bhavasar, S.N., Goswami, R.P. & Evans, G.W. (1993): The Concept of Stress in the Indian tradition. *University of Poona, Publication No. 5, January, Pune.*

Paul, G.L. (1969): Physiological effects of relaxation training and hypnotic suggestion. *Journal for abnormal Psychology, 74, 425-437.*

Pavlov, I.P. (1947): Complete Collection of Works, IV, 351, Moscow-Leningrad, USSR (in Russian, citation as Sokolov, 1963).

Peng, C. K., Mietus, J.E., Liu, Y., Khalsa, G., Douglas, P.S., Benson, H. & Goldberger, A.L. (1998): Exaggerated heart rate oscillations during two meditation techniques. *International Journal of Cardiology*, 70, 101-107.

Pennebaker, J.W. (1982): The Psychology of Physical Symptoms. New York, Springer.

Perez, M.N., Fernandez, M.C., Leon, A.G., Turpin, G. & Vila, J. (1999): Individual Differences associated with Cardiac Defence Response: Psychophysiological and Personality Variables.

Peveler, R.C. & Johnston, D. (1986): Subjective and cognitive effects of relaxation. *Behaviour, Research and Therapy,* 24, (4), 413-419.

Pritchard, R.M. (1961): Stabilized Images on the Retina. *Scientific American*, June 1961.

Puente, A.E & Beiman, I. (1980): The effects of behavior therapy, self-relaxation, and transcendental meditation on cardiovascular stress-response. *Journal of Clinical Psychology, 36, 291 - 295*

Raghuraj, P., Nagarathna, R., Nagendra, H.R. & Telles, S. (1997): Pranayama increases grip strength without lateralized effets. *Indian Journal of Physiology & Pharmacology. 41, 2, 129-133.*

Raju, P.S., Madhavi, S., Prasad, K.V., Reddy, M.E. Sahay, B.K. & Murty, K.J. (1994): Comparison of effects of yoga & physical exercise in atheletes. *Indian Journal of Medical Research. 100, 81-86.*

Ramakrishna, R. (1989): Meditation - secular and sacred, *Journal Indian Academy of Applied Psychology, 15, July, 51-74.*

Reinking, R.H. & Kohl, M.L.(1975): Effects of various forms of relaxation training on physiological and self-report measures of relaxation. *Journal for consulting clinical Psychology 43, 595-600.*

Reyes del Paso, G.A. & Vila J. (1993): Respiratory influences on the cardiac defense response. *International Jouranl of Psychophysiology, 15, 15-26.*

Reyes, G.A., Godoy, J. & Vila, J. (1993): Respiratory sinus arrhythmia as an index of parasympathetic cardiac control during the cardiac defense response. Biological Psychology, 35, 17-35.

Richards, M. & Eves, F., (1991): Personality, Temperament and the Cardiac Defense Response, *Personality and Individual Differencs, 12, 999-1007.*

Richards, M. (1986): Relationships between the Eysenck Personality Questionnaire, Strelau Temperament Inventory and Freiburger Beschwerdenliste Gesamtform, *Personality & Individual Differences, 7, 587-589.*

Sachdeva, U. (1994): The effect of yogic lifestyle on hypertension. *Homeostasis in Health & disease, 35 (4-5), 264-265.*

Sartory, G., Eves. F., & Foa, E. (1989): Maintenance of within session habituation of the cardiac response to phobic stimulation, *Journal of Psychophysiology, 1, 21-34.*

Sawada, Y. & Steptoe, A., (1988): The effects of brief meditation training on cardiovascular stress-responses, *Journal of Psychophysiology, 2 (4), 249 - 257.*

Schalling, D., Cronholm, B. & Asberg, M (1975): Components of state and trait anxiety as related to personality and arousal. In *Emotions: Their parameters and and measurement* (ed. L. Levi), 603-617, Raven Press, New York.

Schandler, S.L. & Grings, W.W. (1976): An examination of methods for producing relaxation during short-term laboratory sessions. *Behavior, Research & Therapy, 14, 419-426.*

Schandry, R.(1989): Lehrbuch der Psychophysiologie, Munich.

Scheider, J.A., Allen, R.A., Agras, W.S., Taylor, C.B. & Southam, M.A. (1980): Stanford Behavioral Medicine Relaxation Procedure, unpublished manual, Stanford CA, USA.

Schmidt, T.F., Wijga, A.H., Robra, B.P., Mueller, M.J. et al. (1994): Yoga training and vegetarian nutrition reduce cardiovascular risk factors in healthy europeans. *Homeostasis in Health & Disease, 35 (4-5), 209-225.*

Schmidt, T.F., Wijga, A.H., Robra, B.P., Mueller, M.J. et al. (1995): Yoga training and vegetarian nutrition reduce cardiovascular risk factors in healthy Europeans: Correction. *Homeostasis in Health & Disease, 36 (2-3), 66.*

Schramm, L., Honig, B., & Bignall, K. (1971): Active muscle vasodilatation in primates homologous with sympathetic vasodilatation in carnivores. *American Journal of Physiology*, 221, 768-777.

Schwartz, G., Davidson, R. & Goleman, D.(1978): Patterning of cognitive and somatic processes in the self-regulation of anxiety: effects of meditation versus exercise. *Psychosomatic Medicine, 40, 321-328.*

Sethi, B.B. & Tiwari, S.C. (1990): Treatment of Anxiety States in India. In: *Anxiety – Psychobiological and Clinical Perspectives,* (eds. N. Sartorius, V. Andreoli, G. Cassano, L. Eisenberg, P., Kielholz, P.Pancheri, G. Racagni) 227-243, Hemisphere P.C. Taylor & Francis, New York.

Shafii, M., Lavely, R.A. & Jaffe, R.D. (1975): Meditation and the prevention of alcohol abuse. *American Journal of Psychiatry, 132, 942-945.*

Shafii, M., Lavely, R.A. & Jaffe, R.D. (1976): Verminderung von Zigarettenrauchen als Folge transzendentaler Meditation [Decrease of Smoking following transcendental meditation]. *Maharishi European Research University Journal*, 24, 29.

Shapiro, D.H. (1985): Clinical use of Meditation as Self-Regulation Strategy. Comments on Holmes Conclusions and Implications. *American Psychologist.* 40, 719-722.

Smith, J.C. (1987): Meditation as psychotherapy: a new look at the evidence. In: *The Psychology of Meditation* (Ed. M. A. West), 136-149, Oxford: Clarendon Press.

Sokolov, E. N. (1963): Higher Nervous functions: The Orienting Reflex. *Annual Review of Physiology, 25, 545-580.*

Spicuzza, L., Gabutti, A., Porta, C., Montano, N., Bernardi, L. (2000): Yoga practice decreases chemoreflex response to hypoxia and hypercapnia. *Lancet 356, 1495-1496.*

Spielberger, C.D., Gorsuch, R.L., Lushene, R., Vagg, P.R. & Jacobs, G.A. (1968, 1977): Self-Evaluation Questionnaire, STAI, Form Y-2. Palo Alto, CA.

Stelmack, R. & Geen, R., 1992: The Psychophysiology of *Extraversion.* In *Handbook of Individual Differences: Biological Perspectives* (eds. A. Gale, & M.W. Eysenck,) Chichester.

Stelmack, R., Kruidenier, B., & Anthony, S., (1985): A factor analysis of the Eysenck Personality Questionnaire and the Strelau Temperament Inventory. *Personality & Individual Differences, 7,* 657-659.

Steptoe, A. (1989): Psychophysiological Interventions in Behavioural Medicine. In *Handbook of Clinical Psychophysiology* (ed. G. Turpin.), John Wiley & Sons Ltd, London.

Strelau, J. (1987): Personality Dimensions based on Arousal Theories: Search for Integration. In J. Strelau, H.J. Eysenck *(eds.)*: Personality Dimensions and Arousal, Plenum Press, New York and London.

Strelau, J. (1990): Introduction: Current Studies on Anxiety from the Perspective Of Research Conducted During the Last Three Decades. In *Anxiety: Recent Developments in Cognitive, Psychophysiological and Health Research* (eds. D. Fogays, T. Sosnowski, K. Wrzesniewski), 1-9, London, Hemisphere PC.

Strelau, J., (1983): Temperament - Personality - Activity, Academic Press, New York.

Strelau, J., Sosnowski, T. & Oniszeszenko, W. (1986): Dynamics of psycho-physiological Changes under Hypoxia and Sensory Deprivation in Subjects with Different Reactivity and Anxiety Levels. In *The biological basis of personality and behaviour,* (eds. J. Strelau, F. Farley & A. Gale,*), 2, 107-116,* London, Hemisphere P.C.

Surwit, R.S. &Williams (Jr.), R.B. & Shapiro, D. (1982): Behavioural approaches to cardiovascular disease, Chapter 3: Introduction to Cardiovascular Psychophysiology, 23-55. Academic Press, New York London,

També, B.V. (1998[2]): Living Meditation through Aum Swarupa. Published by Aum Swarupa, a Learning and Living Community, 1170/12 Revenue Colony, Pune, 411005 India.

Telles, S. & Desiraju, T. (1991): Oxygen consumption during pranayamic type of very slow-rate breathing. *Indian Journal of Medical Research, 94, 357-63.*

Turner, J.R. (1994): Cardiovascular Reactivity and Stress – Patterns of Physiological Response. Plenum Press, New York and London.

Turpin, G. & Siddle, D.A.,(1978): Cardiac and forearm plethysmographic responses to high intensity auditory stimulation. *Biological Psychology, 6, 267 - 281.*

Turpin, G. (1983): Unconditional reflexes and the autonomic nervous system. In: (ed. Siddle, D.A.T.), *Orienting and Habituation*, Wiley, Chichester, 1-70.

Van den Berg, W. & Mulder (1976): Psychological Research on the effects of the transcendental meditation technique on a number of personality variables (Abstract). *Gedrag, Tijdschrift voor Psychologie, 4, 206-218.*

Van Toller, C. (1979): The Nervous Body – An Introduction to the Autonomic Nervous System and Behaviour. Chichester, Wiley.

References

Wallace, R.K. (1970): Physiological effects of transcendental meditation, *Science,* 167, pp 1751-54.

Wallace, R.K., & Benson, H., (1972): The physiology of meditation, *Scientific American,* 226 (2), 84-90.

Walsh, J., Wilding, J. & Eysenck, M. (1993): Stress Responsivity: The Role of Individual Differences. *Personality and Individual Differences, 16, 3, 385-394.*

Wenger, M.A. & Bagchi, B.K. (1961): Studies of autonomic functions in practitioners of Yoga in India, *Behavioural Sciences, 6:* 312-323.

Wenger, M.A. (1941): The measurement of individual differences in autonomic balance. *Psychosomatic Medicine, 3, 334-427.*

Wenger, M.A. (1962): Some problems in psychophysiological research. In: (eds. R. Roessler & N.S. Greenfield) *Physiological correlates of psychological disorder,* 97-114, Wisconsin Press, Madison.

West, M. (1985): Meditation and somatic arousal reduction, *American Psychologist, 40, 717-719.*

West, M. A. (ed.) (1987): The Psychology of Meditation, Oxford: Clarendon Press.

West, M.A. (1980): Meditation, personality and arousal. *Personality and Individual Differences, 1, 135-42.*

Williams, P., Francis, A. & Durham, R. (1976): Personality & Meditation. *Perceptual and Motor Skills, 43, 787-92.*

Winer, B.J. (1971): Statistical principles in experimental design. New York: McGraw-Hill.

Wolfe, J. M. (1994). Guided Search 2.0. A Revised Model of Visual Search. *Psychonomic Bulletin & Review, 1,* 202-238.

Wood, D. (1994): Mood change and perceptions of vitality: a comparison of the effects of relaxation, visualization and yoga. *Journal of the Royal Society of Medicine,* 86 (5), 254-257.

Yardi, N. (2001): Yoga for control of epilepsy. *Seizure-European Journal of Epilepsy, 10, 1, pp.7-12.*